CW00520180

SLOW COOKER DIET

COOKBOOK

Secret and Innovative Recipes to Discover All
You Need to Know About Your Slow Cooker

The Bright Kitchen

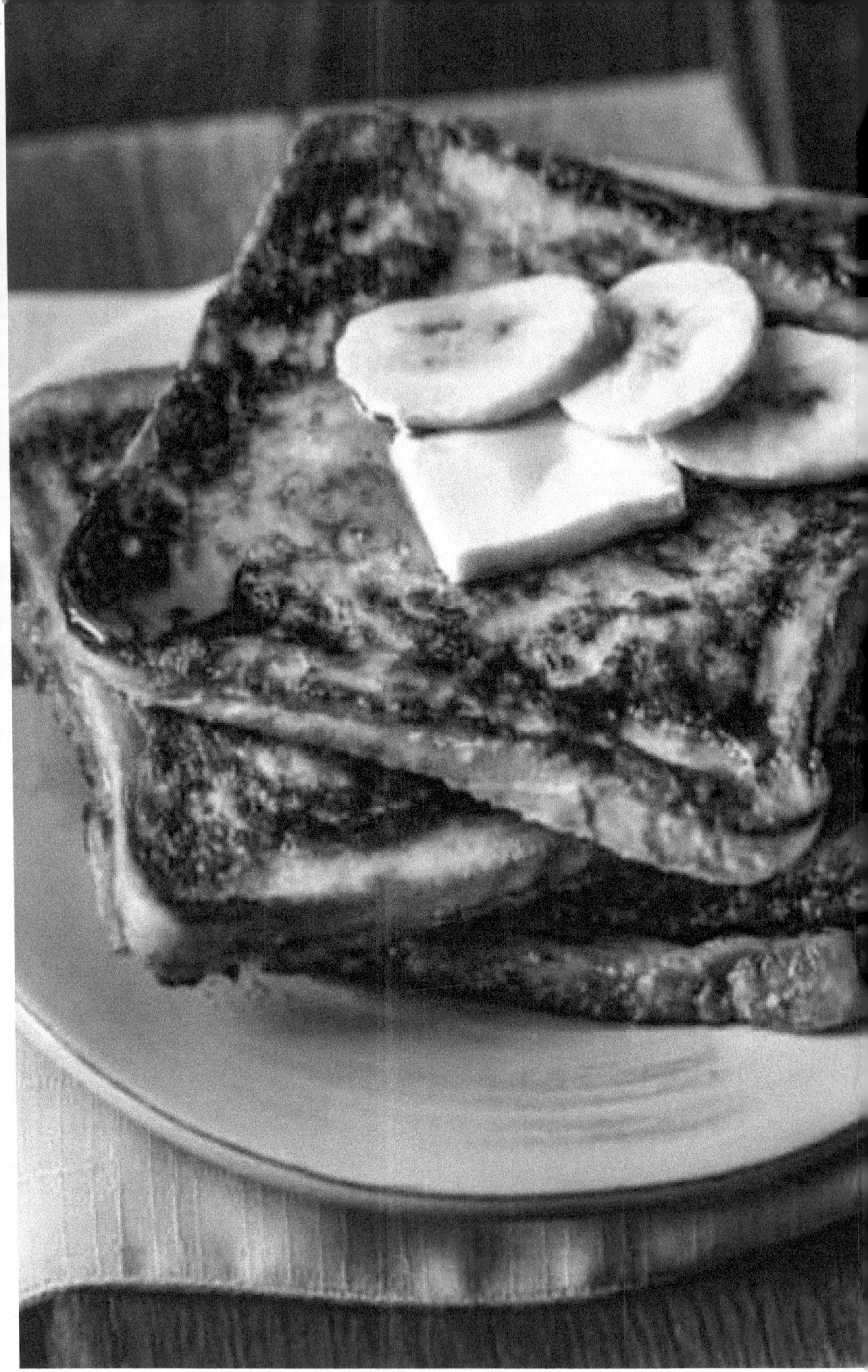

© Copyright 2021 by The Bright Kitchen- All rights reserved.

The following Book is reproduced below with the goal of providing information that is as accurate and reliable as possible. Regardless, purchasing this Book can be seen as consent to the fact that both the publisher and the author of this book are in no way experts on the topics discussed within and that any recommendations or suggestions that are made herein are for entertainment purposes only. Professionals should be consulted as needed prior to undertaking any of the action endorsed herein.

This declaration is deemed fair and valid by both the American Bar Association and the Committee of Publishers Association and is legally binding throughout the United States.

Furthermore, the transmission, duplication, or reproduction of any of the following work including specific information will be considered an illegal act irrespective of if it is done electronically or in print. This extends to creating a secondary or tertiary copy of the work or a recorded copy and is only allowed with the express written consent from the Publisher. All additional right reserved.

The information in the following pages is broadly considered a truthful and accurate account of facts and as such, any inattention, use, or misuse of the information in question by the reader will render any resulting actions solely under their purview. There are no scenarios in which the publisher or the original author of this work can be in any fashion deemed liable for any hardship or damages that may befall them after undertaking information described herein.

Additionally, the information in the following pages is intended only for informational purposes and should thus be thought of as universal. As befitting its nature, it is presented without assurance regarding its prolonged validity or interim quality. Trademarks that are mentioned are done without written consent and can in no way be considered an endorsement from the trademark holder.

Table of Contents

INTRODUCTION

Slow Cooker Cooking

No matter how busy your afternoons or evenings are, a slow cooker allows you to cook more at home and get family meals on the table according to your schedule. Up your meal game by using a slow cooker and elevate your meals from good to great.

A slow cooker, also called a crockpot, is a great appliance that not only produces tasty slow cooker recipes but also saves money and time in the kitchen. You can use your slow cooker to make beef, chicken, lamb and many other meaty recipes, as well as cakes and desserts.

The slow cooker gets its name from the time it needs to cook meals at low temperatures. This is different from a pressure cooker, like an Instant Pot, which uses intense pressure and a short amount of time.

Though times vary, most slow cooker recipes call for cooking on low for eight hours. However, you won't be actively working on the meal during that time. The amount of time you spend preparing your meal is much shorter.

To those in the know, slow cooking breakfast, lunch, dinner, potluck, or dessert recipes is an art form. There's so much more to slow cooking than "setting and forgetting" a few ingredients or a hunk of meat and a package of store-bought slow cooker sauce. Yes, one of the benefits of slow cooking is to prepare ahead time and come home to a fully-cooked big family meal, but a whole world of flavor can be explored with the humble slow cooker.

For some of us, cooking meals every day can seem like a chore. If you don't enjoy spending time leafing through recipes in the kitchen, you're not alone. According to research by Yougov, one in eight of us avoids cooking from scratch.

But when you get things right, slow cooker can be a busy person's best friend, — saving you time and effort. You just need to make sure you don't put the wrong things into your recipe, as this can be a disaster!

How to Use a Slow Cooker

Here are the most basic steps to use a slow cooker:

Prep your ingredients.

1. Add your ingredients to the pot.
2. Put the lid in place.
3. Select your preferred heating level.
4. Set a timer (if necessary) and go about your day.
5. Once the time is up, carefully open the lid and enjoy your meal.

Foods You Can Cook in a Slow Cooker:

- Jams
- Broths
- Desserts
- Meat and poultry
- Beans
- Stuffing
- Porridge
- Fish
- Vegetables
- Soups
- Corn

Things You Shouldn't Put in Your Slow Cooker

Slow cookers are great, but they can't cook everything.

- Dairy
- Too much booze
- Meat that has the skin on
- Lean meats
- Seafood
- Pasta and rice
- Too much spice
- Too much liquid
- Delicate vegetables
- Soft fresh herbs

Important Slow Cooker Tips You Should Know

1. In many cases, the juices left in the pot are like liquid gold. Consider serving them as a sauce or gravy. Use a slurry to thicken it up. A slurry consists of 1 part cornstarch to 2 parts cold water. Start with small amounts and slowly whisk more in until it thickens.

2. If the idea of getting up early to prep your ingredients before heading to work sounds unappealing, you can prep them the night before and store them in the pot in the refrigerator. Then in the morning, you can just take it out, put it in the base, and start cooking.

3. Since some ingredients may cook at different speeds, you might want to stagger the ingredients you add. For instance, I like to wait until the final three hours of a low-temp cook to add potatoes and carrots to a roast. Dairy products are best added at the end.

4. Your slow cooker can do more than just make a one-pot meal. It can be used to keep items warm at potlucks, parties, and other events. A friend of mine uses his crockpot to make large batches of hot chocolate during holiday parties. Scoop it into your mug and add your holiday cheer of choice from the bar.

5. Many slow cooker and Instant Pot recipes are interchangeable. If a meal takes an hour in the Instant

Pot on high pressure, count on it taking eight hours in the slow cooker on low.

6. Be careful to not overfill or under-fill your slow cooker. When learning how to use your slow cooker, one of the top rules is to put the correct amount of food and liquid in the pot.

7. Read the slow cooker manual, and when first using the appliance, take notes of how long your favorite dishes take to cook. Because all crockpots are different, the cooking times can vary.

BREAKFAST

Tasty Bacon Tater

Servings: 8

Preparation Time: 8 hours

Per Serving: Calories: 614 Fat: 36g Carbohydrates: 36.6g

Ingredients:

- 1 Pound Canadian bacon, diced
- 1/2 Cup Parmesan cheese, grated
- 1 Cup whole milk
- Salt and black pepper, to taste
- 1 Pound package frozen tater tot potatoes
- 4 Onions, chopped
- 3 Cups Cheddar cheese, shredded
- 12 Eggs
- 4 Tablespoons flour

Procedure:

1. Firstly, grease a crockpot and layer 1/3 of the tater tots, bacon, onions, and cheeses.
2. Then, repeat the layers twice, ending with cheeses.

3. Mix together eggs, milk, flour, salt and black pepper in a medium mixing bowl.
4. Now, drizzle this mixture over the layers in the crockpot and cover the lid.
5. Finally, cook on LOW about for 8 hours and dish out to serve.

Easy Overnight Quinoa and Oats

Servings: 12

Preparation Time: 4 hours

Per Serving: Calories: 290 Fat: 6g Carbs: 41g

Ingredients:

- 3 Cups steel cut oats no substitutes
- 1 Cup quinoa
- 9 Cups water or almond milk
- 8 Tablespoons brown sugar
- 4 Tablespoons real maple syrup
- 1/2 Teaspoon salt
- 3 Teaspoons vanilla extract
- Optional: 1/4 teaspoon ground cinnamon, fresh berries, splash of milk, additional sugar for topping

Procedure:

1. Firstly, spray your slow cooker with non-stick spray. (Do not forget this step!)
2. In a mesh strainer, rinse the quinoa really well.

3. Then, combine the steel cut outs, rinsed quinoa, water or almond milk, brown sugar, maple syrup, salt, vanilla extract, and cinnamon (if desired) into the slow cooker.

4. Stir really well and then set your slow cooker to low or, if you have a programmable slow cooker, set it to when you will wake up.

5. This meal is ideal at 6-7 hours (best at 6 hours if you have a fast crockpot) and after that it becomes mushy and not so great.

6. If you sleep 6-7 hours then turn it on low right before going to sleep or set the program to start preferably 6 hours before waking up.

7. Now, once you wake up, immediately turn it off the heat and transfer to another dish or to breakfast bowls.

8. Finally, serve with a splash of milk, fresh berries, and additional brown sugar if desired.

Delicious Peach and Blueberry Oatmeal

Servings: 12

Preparation Time: 8 hours

Per Serving: Calories: 172 Fat: 6g Carbs: 30g

Ingredients:

- 6 Cups steel cut oats do not use regular oatmeal because it does not hold up well for slow cooking
- 16 Cups water
- 1 Pound frozen or fresh peaches unsweeetened
- 4 cups frozen blueberries
- 2 Tablespoons real vanilla
- 4 Teaspoons ground cinnamon
- 3 Teaspoons sea salt

Procedure:

1. Firstly, spray slow cooker with cooking spray or use a crockpot liner.
2. Combine all of the ingredients in the crockpot.
3. The cinnamon and fruit will probably rise to the top, don't worry about it. They will cook up just fine.
4. Then, cook overnight on low for 8 hours.
5. Now, serve with sweetener of choice, butter or milk.

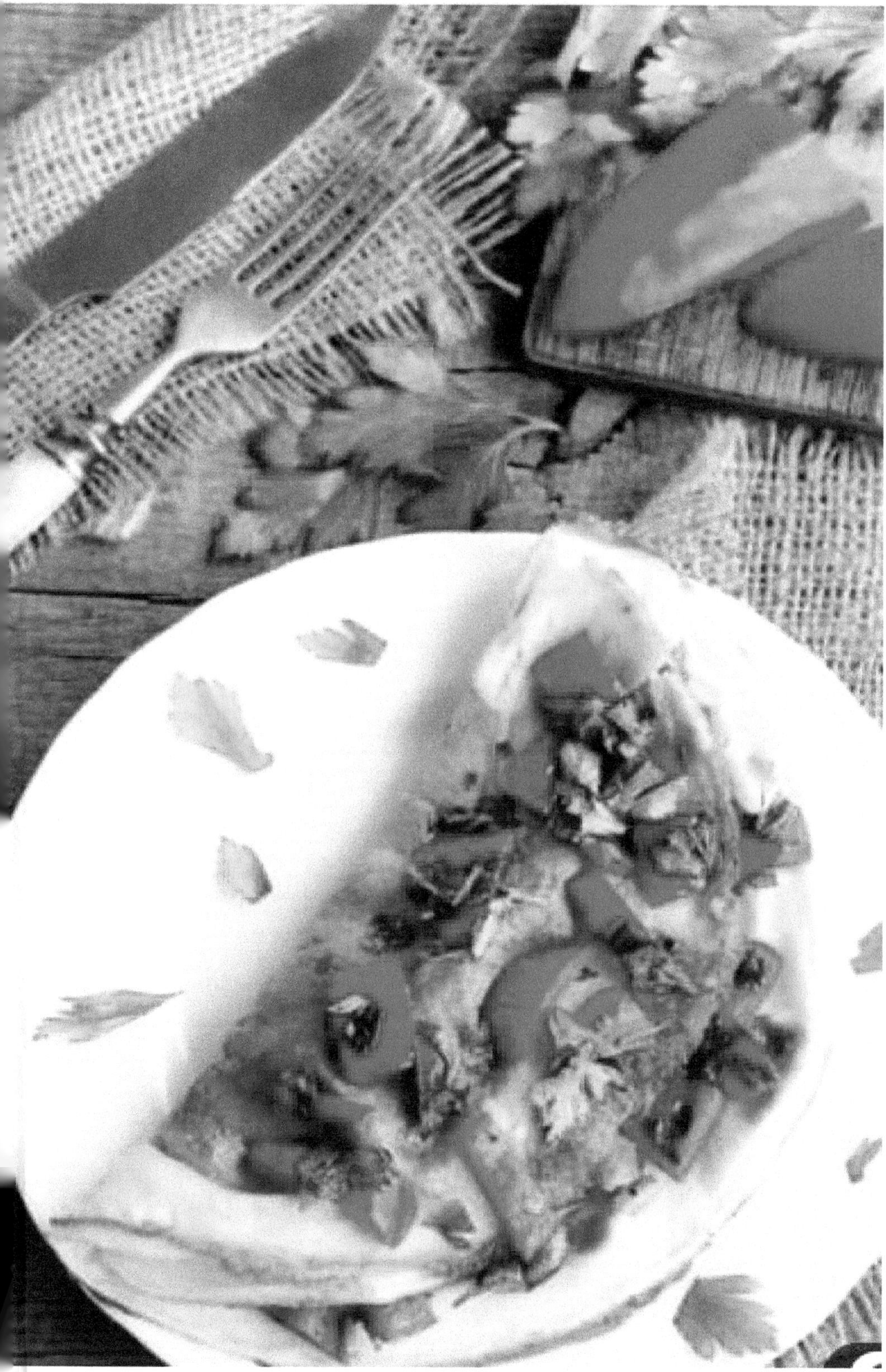

Tempting Vegetable Omelette

Servings: 12

Preparation Time: 2 hours

Per Serving: Calories: 144 Fat: 7g Carbs: 8g

Ingredients:

- 12 Eggs
- 1 Cup milk
- 1/2 Teaspoon salt
- Fresh ground pepper, to taste
- 1/4 Teaspoon garlic powder, or to taste
- 1/4 Teaspoon chili powder, or to taste
- 1 Cup broccoli florets
- 2 Red bell peppers, thinly sliced
- 2 Small yellow onions, finely chopped
- 2 Garlic cloves, minced
- Garnish
- Shredded cheddar cheese
- Chopped tomatoes
- Chopped onions
- Fresh parsley

Procedure:

1. Firstly, lightly grease the inside of the slow cooker/crock pot with cooking spray; set aside.
2. Then, in a large mixing bowl combine eggs, milk, salt, pepper, garlic powder and chili powder; using egg beaters or a whisk, beat the mixture until mixed and well combined.
3. Add broccoli florets, sliced peppers, onions and garlic to the slow cooker; stir in the egg-mixture.
4. Now, cover and cook on HIGH for 2 hours. Start checking at 1 hour 30 minutes. Omelette is done when eggs are set.
5. Sprinkle with cheese and cover; let stand 2 to 3 minutes or until cheese is melted.
6. Turn off the slow cooker.
7. Cut the omelette into 8 wedges.
8. Transfer to a serving plate.
9. Garnish with chopped tomatoes, chopped onions and fresh parsley.
10. Finally, serve.

Enticing Quinoa Breakfast Casserole

Servings: 8

Preparation Time: 4 hours

Per Serving: Calories: 270 Fat: 12g Carbs: 20g

Ingredients:

- 1 Cup quinoa rinsed well and uncooked
- 3 Cups milk (I used 2%)
- 12 Large eggs
- 1 Teaspoon salt
- 1/4 Teaspoon pepper
- 1 Cup frozen cut leaf spinach or use a handful of fresh!
- 3/4 Cup grape tomatoes halved
- 1/2 Cup shredded cheese colby, monterey jack, cheddar, etc.
- 1/2 Cup shredded Parmesan cheese

Procedure:

1. Firstly, in a mixing bowl whisk 6 eggs until beaten.
2. Then, add quinoa, milk, salt and pepper and whisk until combined.

3. Gently mix in spinach, tomatoes and 1/2 cup shredded cheese
4. Spray crock well with nonstick spray
5. Add egg and quinoa mixture to crock
6. Now, top with Parmesan cheese
7. Finally, cover and cook on high for 2-4 hours until eggs are set and edges are lightly browned

Delectable Cauliflower Hash Brown

Servings: 8

Preparation Time: 5 hours

Per Serving: Calories: 131 Fat: 10g Carbs: 6g

Ingredients:

- 24 Eggs
- 1 Cup milk
- 1 Teaspoon dry mustard
- 2 Teaspoons kosher salt
- 1 Teaspoon pepper
- 2 Heads cauliflower shredded
- Additional salt and pepper to season the layers
- Up to one small onion diced (can omit or use less)
- Two 5 oz packages pre-cooked breakfast sausages sliced (I used turkey sausage.
- Can also omit, or use about 1 lb bulk breakfast sausage cooked and crumbled, or bacon, vegetarian sausage crumbles, or chopped ham)
- 16 Oz. or about 2 cups shredded cheddar cheese

Procedure:

1. Firstly, grease or coat a 6 quart slow cooker with cooking spray.
2. Lightly beat together the eggs, milk, dry mustard, salt, and pepper.
3. Then, place about a third of the shredded cauliflower in an even layer in the bottom of the slow cooker, and top with about a third of the onion.
4. Season with salt and pepper, the top with about a third of the sausage and a third of the cheese. Repeat the layers two more times.
5. Now, pour the egg mixture over the contents of the slow cooker.
6. Finally, cook on a low heat for 5-7 hours, or until eggs are set and the top is browned.

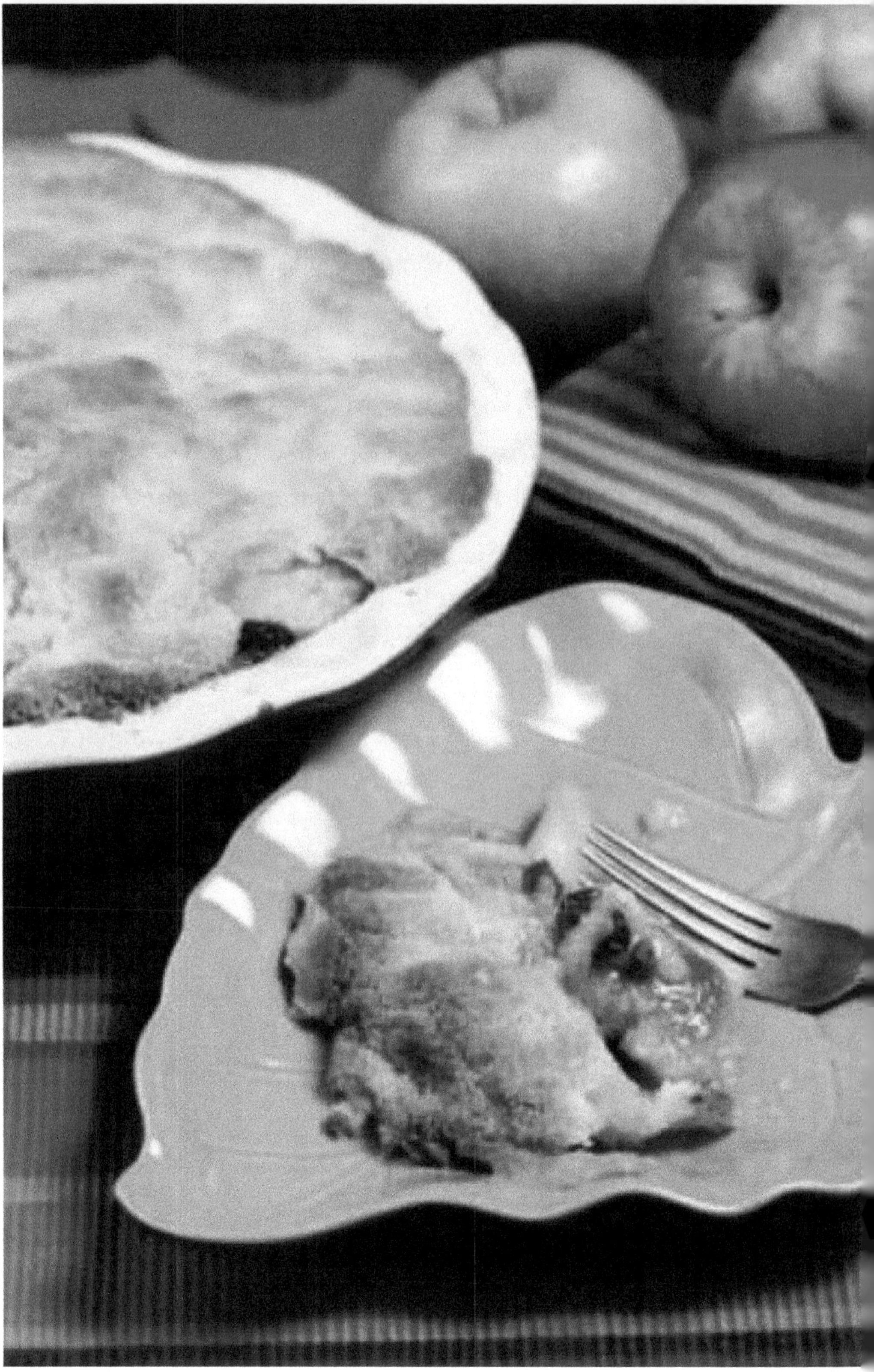

Delightful Apple Cobbler

Servings: 4

Preparation Time: 3 hours

Ingredients:

- 4 Medium, tart apples
- 1/4 Cup sugar
- 1 Tablespoon fresh lemon juice
- 1 Teaspoon lemon zest
- Dash of ground cinnamon
- 1 Cup natural fat-free cereal mixed with fruit and nuts
- 1/8 Cup butter, melted
- Cooking spray

Procedure:

1. Fistly, spritz the slow cooker lightly with cooking spray.
2. Core, peel, and slice apples into the slow cooker.
3. Then, add sugar, lemon juice and zest, and cinnamon.
4. Mix cereal and melted butter together, then add to the ingredients in the slow cooker. Mix thoroughly.
5. Now, cook on low for 6 hours or on high for 2 to 3 hours.
6. Finally, serve warm.

Easy Eggs in Tomato Purgatory

Servings: 4

Preparation Time: 8 hours

Ingredients:

- 1 Pound (1.1 kg) Roma tomatoes, chopped
- 1 Onion, chopped
- 1 Garlic clove, chopped
- 1/2 Teaspoon paprika
- 1/4 Teaspoon ground cumin
- 1/4 Teaspoon dried marjoram leaves
- 1/2 Cup vegetable broth
- 4 Large eggs
- 1 Red chili peppers, minced
- 1/4 Cup chopped flat-leaf parsley

Procedure:

1. Firstly, in the slow cooker, mix the tomatoes, onions, garlic, paprika, cumin, marjoram, and vegetable broth, and stir to mix.
2. Then, cover and cook on low for 7 to 8 hours, or until a sauce has formed.

3. One at a time, break the eggs into the sauce, then do not stir.
4. Cover and cook on high until the egg whites are completely set and the yolk is thickened, about 20 minutes.
5. Sprinkle the eggs with the minced red chili peppers.
6. Now, sprinkle with the parsley and serve.

Tasty Potato and Tomato Strata

Servings: 4

Preparation Time: 8 hours

Ingredients:

- 4 Yukon Gold potatoes, peeled and diced
- 1/2 Onion, minced
- 1 red bell peppers, stemmed, deseeded, and minced
- 1.1/2 Roma tomatoes, deseeded and chopped
- 1 Garlic cloves, minced
- 1 Cup shredded Swiss cheese
- 4 Eggs
- 1 Egg whites
- 1/2 Teaspoon dried marjoram leaves
- 1 Cup 2% milk

Procedure:

1. Firstly, in the slow cooker, layer the diced potatoes, onion, bell peppers, tomatoes, garlic, and cheese.
2. In a medium bowl, mix the eggs, egg whites, marjoram, and milk well with a wire whisk.
3. Then, pour this mixture into the slow cooker.

4. Now, cover and cook on low for 6 to 8 hours, or until a food thermometer inserted in the mixture registers 165ºF (74ºC) and the potatoes are tender.
5. Finally, scoop out of the slow cooker to serve.

Pleasant Banana and Pecan French toast

Servings: 4

Preparation Time: 2 hours

Ingredients:

- 2 Teaspoons butter, at room temperature
- 4 Eggs
- ¾ Cup 2% milk
- 2 Teaspoons vanilla extract
- 2 Teaspoons ground cinnamon
- 1/2 Teaspoon ground nutmeg
- 1/4 Teaspoon sea salt
- 4 Cups sliced bananas
- 8 Slices whole-grain bread, crusts removed, cut into 1-inch cubes
- 4 Tablespoons finely chopped toasted pecans

Procedure:

1. Firstly, grease the slow cooker with the butter.
2. In a large bowl, whisk together the eggs, milk, vanilla, cinnamon, nutmeg, and salt.

3. Then, gently toss the bananas and bread cubes in the mixture until the bread is thoroughly saturated.
4. Pour the bread and banana mixture into the slow cooker. Sprinkle the top with the toasted pecans.
5. Now, cover and cook on low for 4 hours or on high for 2 hours.
6. Finally, serve warm.

Flavorful Morning Muesli

Servings: 12

Preparation Time: 4 hours

Per Serving: 262 calories, 4g protein, 19.8g carbohydrates, 20.3g fat, 4g fiber, 0mg cholesterol, 13mg sodium, 346mg potassium.

Ingredients:

- 2 Cups oatmeal
- 2 Tablespoons raisins
- 2 Teaspoons sesame seeds
- 2 Teaspoons dried cranberries
- 2 Bananas, chopped
- 2 Teaspoons ground cinnamon
- 4 Cups of coconut milk

Procedure:

1. Firstly, mix coconut milk with oatmeal, raisins, sesame seeds, dried cranberries, and ground cinnamon.
2. Transfer the ingredients in the slow cooker and cook on low for 4 hours.

3. Then, stir carefully and transfer in the serving bowls.
4. Now, top the muesli with chopped banana.

Tasty Breakfast Monkey Bread

Servings: 12

Preparation Time: 6 hours

Per Serving: 178 calories, 6.1g protein, 26.4g carbohydrates, 7g fat, 2g fiber, 27mg cholesterol, 238mg sodium, 21mg potassium.

Ingredients:

- 20 Oz biscuit rolls
- 2 Tablespoons ground cardamom
- 2 Tablespoons sugar
- 4 Tablespoons coconut oil
- 2 Eggs, beaten

Procedure:

1. Firstly, chop the biscuit roll roughly.
2. Mix sugar with ground cardamom.
3. Then, melt the coconut oil.
4. Put the ½ part of chopped biscuit rolls in the slow cooker in one layer and sprinkle with melted coconut oil and ½ part of all ground cinnamon mixture.

5. Top it with remaining biscuit roll chops and sprinkle with cardamom mixture and coconut oil.
6. Now, brush the bread with a beaten egg and close the lid.
7. Cook the meal on high for 6 hours.
8. Finally, cook the cooked bread well.

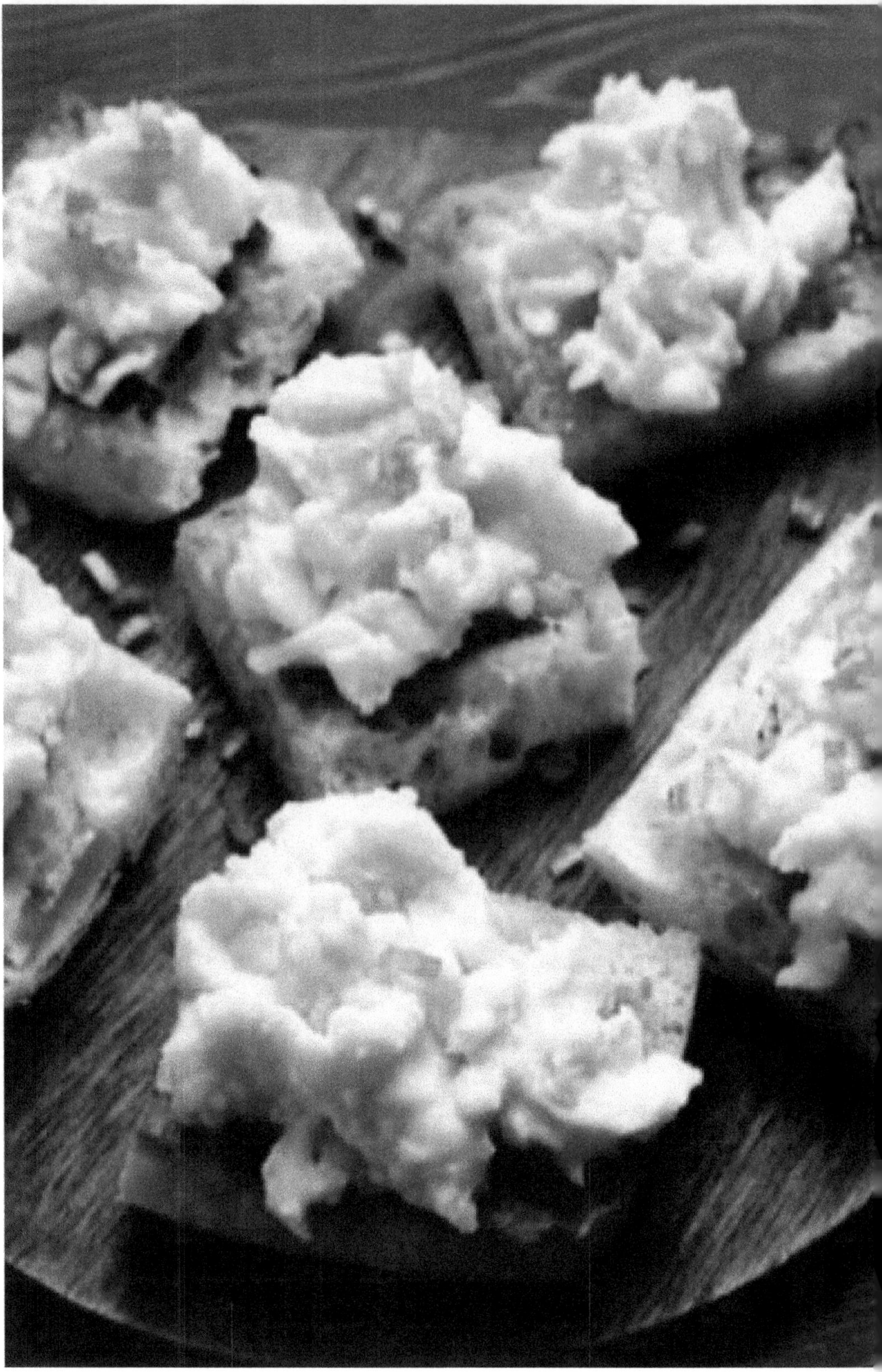

Tempting Egg Scramble

Servings: 8

Preparation Time: 2.5 hours

Per Serving: 147 calories, 9.2g protein, 0.9g carbohydrates, 12g fat, 0.2g fiber, 186mg cholesterol, 170mg sodium, 88mg potassium.

Ingredients:

- 8 Eggs, beaten
- 2 Tablespoons butter, melted
- 24 Oz Cheddar cheese, shredded
- 1/2 Teaspoon cayenne pepper
- 2 Teaspoons ground paprika

Procedure:

1. Firstly, mix eggs with butter, cheese, cayenne pepper, and ground paprika.
2. Then, pour the mixture in the slow cooker and close the lid.

3. Cook it on high for 2 hours.

4. Now, open the lid and scramble the eggs.

5. Finally, close the lid and cook the meal on high for 30 minutes.

LUNCH

Delicious Mediterranean Vegetable Lasagna

Servings: 4

Preparation Time: 6 hours

Per Serving: Calories: 510 Carbohydrate: 21g Fat: 31g

Ingredients:

- 6 Uncooked whole wheat lasagna noodles
- 16 Ounces marinara sauce
- 12 Ounces skim ricotta cheese
- 8 Ounces chopped spinach, frozen and liquid squeezed -
- 6 Ounces mushrooms
- -1 Pound mozzarella cheese
- 3 Ounces cherry tomatoes
- 1/4 Cup chopped fresh parsley
- 1/2 Teaspoon salt

Procedure:

1. Firstly, in a medium bowl, put spinach, ricotta cheese, salt and combine.
2. Then, spread half a cup of tomato sauce into the bottom of a 6-quart slow cooker.

3. Break the noodles and layer a portion of it on the tomato sauce.
4. Now, on top of the noodles, layer ricotta mixture, along with one-third portions of mushrooms, and one-third portions of mozzarella cheese, and a cup of marinara sauce.
5. Above this layer, add another portion of broken noodles.
6. Again layer mozzarella cheese, tomato sauce, and cherry tomatoes.
7. Repeat the layering process until you can make 3 layers.
8. Close the lid and slow cook 6 hours.
9. Once the cooking is over, allow it to settle for 30 minutes.
10. Finally, garnish it with chopped parsley while serving.

Easy Crockpot Tortellini Stew

Servings: 4

Preparation Time: 8 hours

Per Serving: Calories: 170 Carbohydrate: 26g Fat: 3g

Ingredients:

- 1 Medium zucchini cut into one-inch slices
- 1/2 Small finely chopped onion
- 14 Ounces diced tomatoes, undrained -
- 14 Ounces vegetable broth
- 7 Ounces great Northern Beans -
- 1/2 Tablespoon dried basil leaves
- 1/8 Teaspoon pepper
- 4 Ounces uncooked dry cheese filled tortellini
- 1/8 Teaspoon Salt

Procedure:

1. Firstly, put onion, vegetable broth, zucchini, great northern beans, tomatoes, pepper and salt into a 6-quart slow cooker. Combine it thoroughly.
2. Then, close the slow cooker and slow cook for 8 hours.

3. Twenty minutes before serving, stir in tortellini and basil.
4. Now, put on high heat for 20 minutes until the tortellini becomes tender.
5. Finally, serve hot.

Yummy Slow Cooker Spinach lasagna

Servings: 4

Preparation Time: 6.5 hours

Per Serving: Calories: 440 Carbohydrate: 37g Fat: 22g

Ingredients:

- 7 Ounces canned diced tomatoes, undrained
- 14 Ounces organic tomato basil paste sauce
- 1/2 Coarsely chopped yellow bell pepper
- 1/8 Teaspoon red pepper, crushed
- 4 Uncooked lasagna noodles
- 1/2 Thinly sliced zucchini
- 3 Ounces shredded skimmed mozzarella cheese
- 1 Cup light ricotta cheese
- 2 Ounces coarsely chopped fresh baby spinach

Procedure:

1. Firstly, spray some cooking spray in the bottom of a 6-quart slow cooker.
2. In a medium bowl, mix tomatoes, pasta sauce, bell pepper, crushed red pepper, and zucchini.

3. Then, spread a cup of tomato mixture on the bottom part of the slow cooker.

4. Layer the three lasagna noodles over the tomato mixture. Break the noodles so that you can easily layer the noodles.

5. Now, layer half portion of the ricotta cheese on top of the noodles.

6. Sprinkle half the quantity of spinach and 1/4 cup of mozzarella cheese above the layer.

7. Top it with one-third portion of tomato sauce mixture.

8. Repeat the layering process of noodles, cheese, and spinach for at least three layers.

9. Cover the slow cooker and slow cook for 6 hours until the noodles become tender.

10. Before serving, sprinkle mozzarella all over the lasagna and let it the cheese start melting.

Tempting Crockpot Mediterranean Egg Plant Dish

Servings: 4

Preparation Time: 9 hours

Per Serving: Calories: 63 Carbohydrate: 4.1g Fat: 5.2g

Ingredients:

- ½ Diced onion
- 1 Medium peeled and cubed eggplants
- 1/2 Can diced tomatoes
- 1 Diced carrots
- 1.1/2 Tablespoons veg oil
- 1/2 Tablespoon tomato paste
- 1/8 Teaspoon salt
- 1/4 Teaspoon pepper
- Paprika – as required
- Water – as needed
- 1/8 Cup cilantro chopped

Procedure:

1. Firstly, in a large bowl, put cubed eggplants, add water and salt. Stir it so that it can remove the bitter taste of eggplants.
2. Pour oil into a saucepan and bring to medium heat.
3. Then, put the chopped onion and sauté until it turns light brown and keeps it aside.
4. Now, put canned tomatoes, tomato paste, and paprika into a 6-quart slow cooker.
5. Remove the eggplants from the water and wash it under running tap water.
6. Finally, put the eggplants along with the chopped carrots into the slow cooker.
7. Transfer the sautéed onion into the slow cooker and combine all the ingredients.
8. Add a sufficient quantity of water to cook the vegetables or until the eggplants and carrots get entirely immersed.
9. Add pepper and salt as per your taste required.
10. Set slow cooker for 9 hours.
11. Garnish with chopped cilantro before serving.
12. Serve hot with rice and salad.

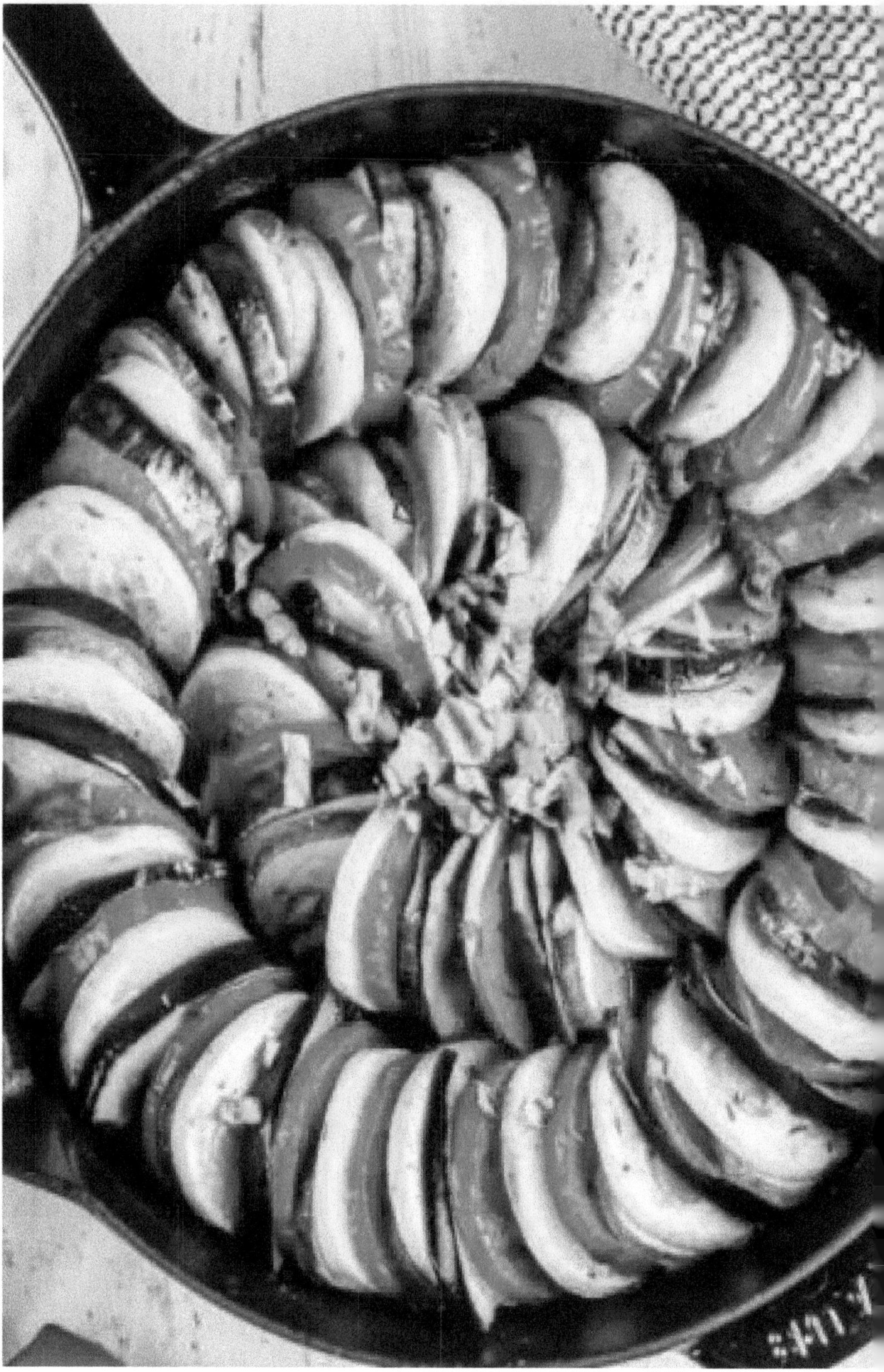

Tasty Slow Cooker Ratatouille

Servings: 12

Preparation Time: 6 hours

Per Serving: Calories: 130 Carbohydrate: 15g Fat: 8g

Ingredients:

- 1 Medium Eggplant, cut into ¾" size
- 4 Tablespoons tomato paste
- 6 Tablespoons olive oil -
- 2 Pounds plum tomatoes, medium dice
- 1/2 Teaspoon freshly ground black pepper
- 2 Large yellow bell peppers cut into ¼ inch slices
- 16 Ounces yellow summer squash, cut into 3/4 inch pieces
- 8 Large cloves garlic, finely sliced
- 1 Bay leaf
- 2 large onions sliced into half
- 2 Tablespoons fresh thyme leaves, chopped
- 3 Teaspoons salt
- Fresh basil leaves, cut in ribbon size - for garnish

Procedure:

1. Firstly, in a large bowl, put eggplant, one teaspoon salt and add water.
2. Stir it and keep it aside. Drain after 30 minutes.
3. Rinse it under running tap water and place the eggplant over a paper towel.
4. Then, take a new bowl and whisk tomato paste, oil and the remaining salt along with black pepper.
5. Now, combine the drained eggplant, zucchini or squash, tomatoes, onion, bell pepper, thyme, garlic in a slow cooker.
6. Add the tomato-oil paste mixture into the slow cooker and combine.
7. Add bay leaf.
8. Cover and slow cook for 4 hours until the vegetable becomes tender.
9. After four hours, open up the lid and cook for one more hour to let the extra liquid evaporate.
10. Discard the bay leaf before serving.
11. Finally, garnish with fresh basil leaves before serving.

Pleasant Garlicky Chicken

Servings: 12

Preparation Time: 6 hours

Ingredients:

- 1/2 Cup dry white wine
- 4 Tablespoons chopped dried parsley
- 4 Teaspoons dried basil leaves
- 1 Teaspoon dried oregano
- Pinch of crushed red pepper flakes
- 40 Cloves of garlic (about 1 head)
- 8 Celery ribs, chopped
- 12 Boneless, skinless chicken breast halves
- 2 Lemons, juiced and zested
- Fresh herbs, for garnish (optional)

Procedure:

1. Firstly, combine the wine, parsley, basil, oregano, and red peppers in a large bowl.
2. Add the garlic cloves and celery to the bowl. Coat well.
3. Then, transfer the garlic and celery to a slow cooker with a slotted spoon.

4. Add the chicken to the spice mixture. Coat well. Place the chicken on top of the vegetables in the slow cooker.

5. Drizzle with the lemon juice and sprinkle with the lemon zest in the slow cooker.

6. Add any remaining spice mixture.

7. Now, cook on low for 5 to 6 hours, or until chicken is no longer pink in center.

8. Finally, garnish with fresh herbs, if desired. Serve warm.

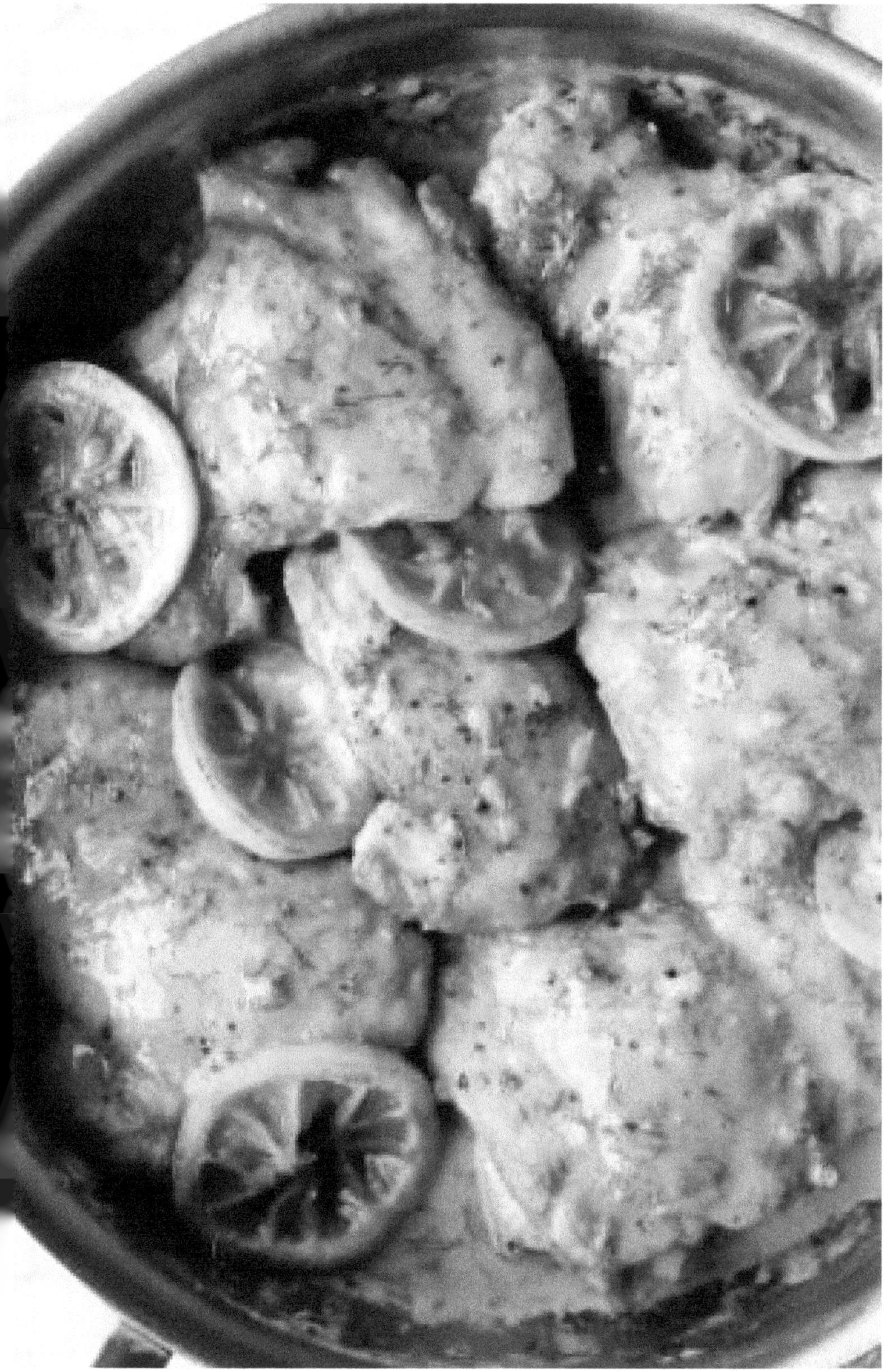

Easy Lemony Dill Chicken

Servings: 8

Preparation Time: 4 hours

Ingredients:

- 2 Cups fat-free sour cream
- 2 Tablespoons fresh dill, minced
- 2 Teaspoons lemon pepper seasoning
- 2 Teaspoons lemon zest
- 4 Boneless, skinless chicken breast halves

Procedure:

1. First, combine the sour cream, dill, lemon pepper, and lemon zest in a small bowl.
2. Then, spoon one-fourth of the sour cream mixture into a slow cooker.
3. Arrange the chicken breasts on top in a single layer.
4. Pour the remaining sauce over the chicken. Spread evenly.
5. Now, cook on low for 3 to 4 hours or until juices run clear.
6. Finally, serve warm.

Easy Toasted Sesame Chicken Wings

Servings: 4

Preparation Time: 5 hours

Ingredients:

- 1.1/2 Pounds (1.4 kg) chicken wings
- Salt, to taste
- Pepper, to taste
- 1 Cup honey
- 1/2 Cup soy sauce
- ¼ Cup ketchup
- 1 Tablespoon canola oil
- 1 Tablespoon sesame oil
- 1 Garlic cloves, minced
- Toasted sesame seeds, for topping

Procedure:

1. First, rinse the wings.
2. Cut at the joint.
3. Sprinkle with salt and pepper.
4. Place on a broiler pan.

5. Broil at 180ºF (82ºC) for 10 minutes on each side. Place the chicken in a slow cooker.
6. Combine the remaining ingredients, except for sesame seeds, in a bowl. Pour over the chicken.
7. Then cover. Cook on low for 5 hours or on high for 2½ hours.
8. Now, sprinkle the sesame seeds over top just before serving.

Yummy Oregano Millet

Servings: 6

Preparation Time: 3 hours

Per Serving: 162 calories, 3.9g protein, 24.9g carbohydrates, 5.2g fat, 3g fiber, 14mg cholesterol, 6mg sodium, 81mg potassium.

Ingredients:

- 1/2 Cup heavy cream
- 1 Cup millet
- 2 Teaspoons dried oregano
- 2 Cups of water

Procedure:

1. Firstly, put all ingredients from the list above in the slow cooker.
2. Then, close the lid and cook on high for 3 hours.

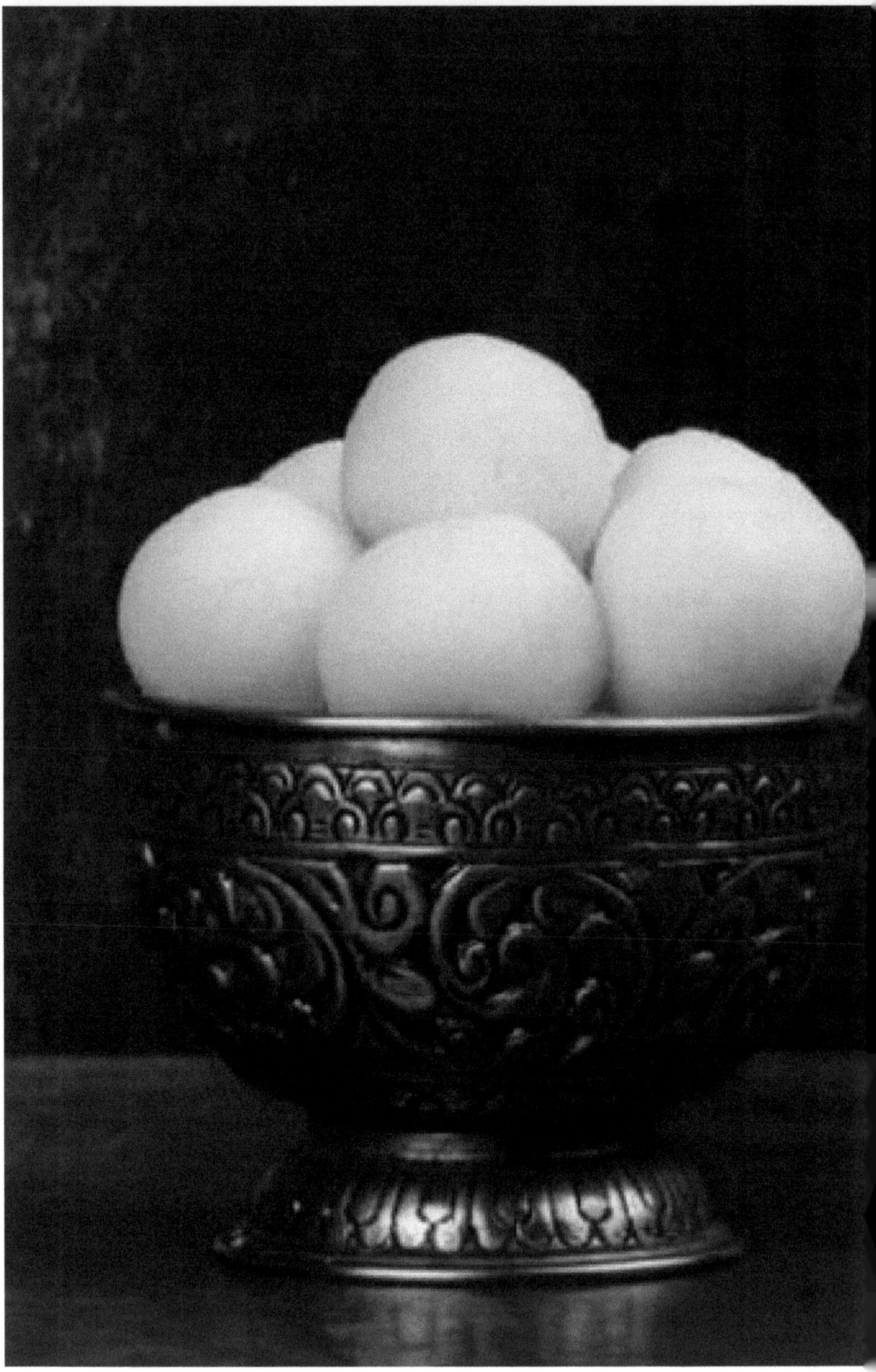

Flavorful Milky Semolina

Servings: 4

Preparation Time: 1 hour

Per Serving: 180 calories, 8.7g protein, 26.5g carbohydrates, 4g fat, 0.8g fiber, 15mg cholesterol, 87mg sodium, 147mg potassium.

Ingredients:

- 1/2 Cup semolina
- 3 Cups milk
- 2 Teaspoons vanilla extract
- 2 Teaspoons sugar

Procedure:

1. Firstly, put all ingredients in the slow cooker.
2. Them, close the lid and cook the semolina on high for 1 hour.
3. When the meal is cooked, carefully stir it and cool it to room temperature.

Easy Rice Boats

Servings: 8

Preparation Time: 2.5 hours

Per Serving: 151 calories, 5.8g protein, 31.6g carbohydrates, 1.7g fat, 11.1g fiber, 3mg cholesterol, 16mg sodium, 734mg potassium.

Ingredients:

- 4 Medium eggplants
- 2 Cups wild rice, cooked
- 2 Teaspoons dried basil
- 1/2 Cup broccoli, shredded
- 2 Teaspoons butter, melted
- 1/2 Teaspoon ground black pepper
- 1/2 Cup of water

Procedure:

1. Firstly, cut the eggplants into halves and remove the flesh.
2. In the mixing bowl, mix rice with basil, broccoli, ground black pepper, and butter.

3. Then, fill the eggplant halves with rice mixture and arrange them in the slow cooker.
4. Add water and close the lid.
5. Finally, cook the rice boats on high for 2.5 hours.

Enticing Tomato Dal

Servings: 12

Preparation Time: 7 hours

Per Serving: 235 calories, 10.9g protein, 45.9g carbohydrates, 0.7g fat, 10.8g fiber, 0mg cholesterol, 12mg sodium, 432mg potassium.

Ingredients:

- 2 Teaspoons scumin seeds
- 1 Cup red lentils
- 1 Teaspoon fennel seeds
- 10 Cups of water
- 1 Cup tomatoes, chopped
- 1/2 Cup onion, diced
- 1 Teaspoon ground ginger
- 2 Cups of rice

Procedure:

1. Firstly, put ingredients from the list above in the slow cooker.
2. Then, carefully stir the mixture and close the lid.
3. Now, cook the tomato dal on low for 7 hours.

Delicious Cherry Rice

Servings: 8

Preparation Time: 3 hours

Per Serving: 249 calories, 3.9g protein, 51.1g carbohydrates, 3.3g fat, 1.4g fiber, 8mg cholesterol, 29mg sodium, 136mg potassium.

Ingredients:

- 2 Cups basmati rice
- 2 Cups cherries, raw
- 6 Cups of water
- 4 Tablespoons of liquid honey
- 2 Tablespoons butter, melted

Procedure:

1. Firstly, put cherries and rice in the slow cooker.
2. Then, add water and cook the meal on high for 3 hours.
3. Meanwhile, mix liquid honey and butter.
4. When the rice is cooked, add liquid honey mixture and carefully stir.

DINNER

Delicious Smoked Sausage and Sauerkraut Soup

Servings: 12

Preparation Time: 5 hours

Per Serving: Calories: 197 Fat: 12g Carbs: 12g

Ingredients:

- 2 lbs smoked sausage sliced
- 8 Large potatoes or 6 - 8 small potatoes, chopped
- 1 Onion chopped
- 30 Oz cans sauerkraut drained and rinsed
- 2 Can diced tomatoes
- 16 Oz tomato sauce
- 64 Oz chicken broth

Procedure:

1. Firstly, place all ingredients in slow cooker and stir.
2. Then, cook on high 5-6 hours or low 7-8 hours.

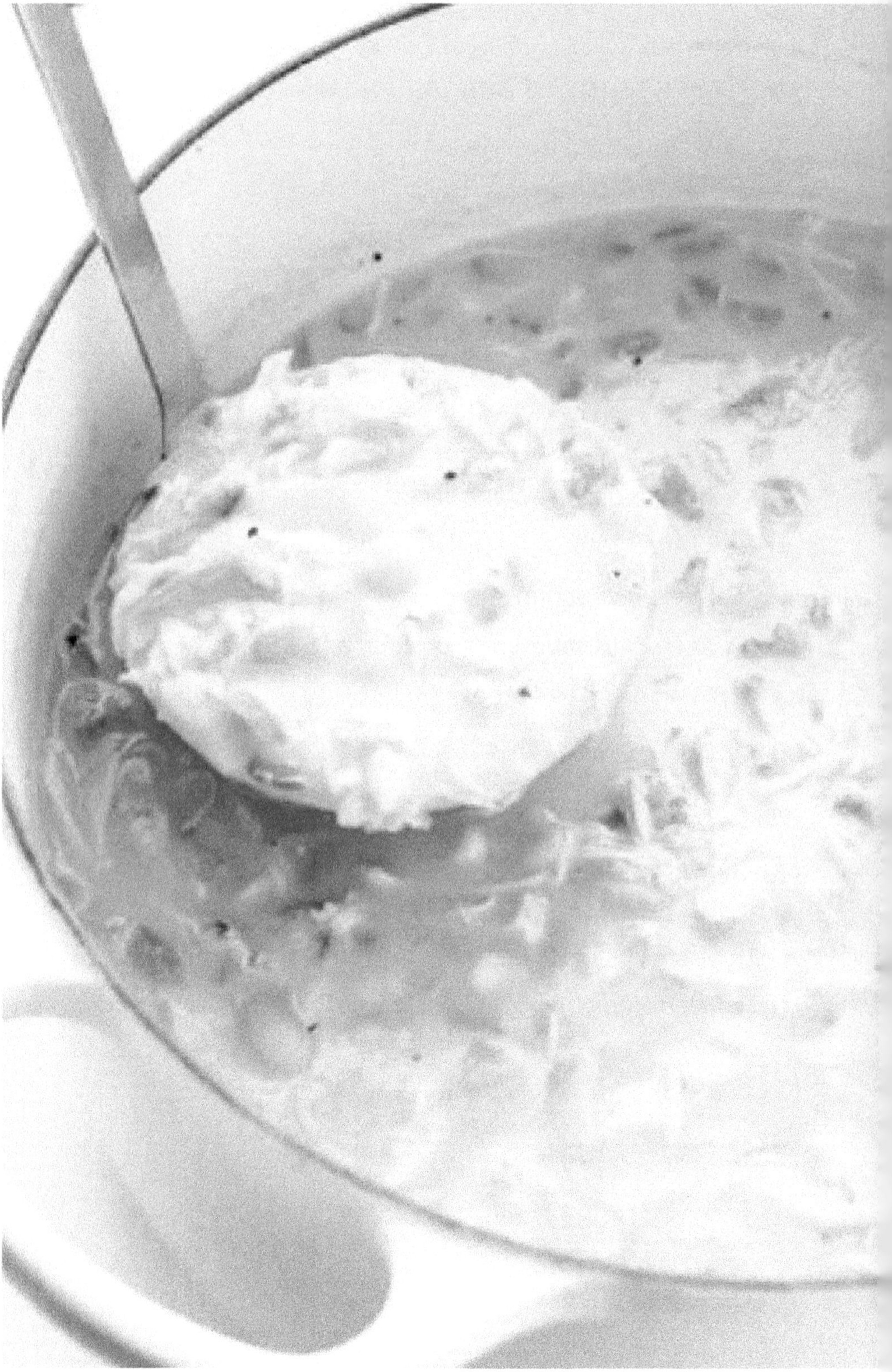

Delectable White Chicken Chili

Servings: 12

Preparation Time: 8 hours

Per Serving: Calories: 176 Fat: 5g Carbs: 20g

Ingredients:

- 5 lbs. bone-in chicken pieces I used 2 very large chicken breasts
- 2 Onions chopped
- 6 Garlic cloves crushed
- 2 Can chopped green chilies
- 2 lbs great northern beans soaked
- 4 Tsps cumin
- 2 Tsps oregano
- 1/4 Tsp. cayenne pepper
- 2 Tsps chili powder
- 64 Oz box chicken broth
- 4 Cups water
- Salt to taste
- 4 Tbsps cornmeal
- 2 Cups milk

Procedure:

1. Firstly, place all ingredients in the slow cooker, except the cornmeal and milk.
2. Then, cook on high 6-7 hours or low 8-9 hours.
3. Remove chicken from soup and shred.
4. Now, return chicken to soup.
5. Stir cornmeal and milk together and add to the soup to thicken.
6. Finally, adjust seasonings and serve.

Tempting Chicken Cock-a-Leekie Soup

Servings: 12

Preparation Time: 5 hours

Per Serving: Calories: 220 Fat: 3g Carbs: 36g

Ingredients:

- 4 Bone-in chicken breasts
- 6 Leeks sliced and cleaned
- 10 Carrots chopped
- 1/3 Cup barley
- 2 Onions chopped
- 1 Bay leaf
- 2 Tsps thyme
- 64 Oz boxes chicken broth
- Salt and pepper to taste
- Dried prunes diced for topping, optional

Procedure:

1. Firstly, place chicken breasts in slow cooker.
2. Then, add leeks, carrots, barley, onion, bay leaf and thyme to slow cooker.

3. Pour chicken broth over all ingredients.

4. Now, cook on high 5-6 hours or low 7-8 hours.

5. Remove chicken breasts and take meat off of bones.

6. Return meat to the soup.

7. Finally, serve with diced prunes.

Easy Farro with Mushrooms

Servings: 12

Preparation Time: 3 hours

Ingredients:

- 4 Shallots, minced
- 1 Ounce (14 g) dried porcini mushrooms, rinsed and minced
- 4 Tablespoons extra-virgin olive oil, divided
- 6 Garlic cloves, minced
- 4 Teaspoons minced fresh thyme or ½ teaspoon dried
- Salt and ground black pepper, to taste
- 5 Cups vegetable or chicken broth, divided, plus extra as needed
- ½ Cup dry sherry
- 16 Ounces (227 g) cremini mushrooms, trimmed and sliced thin
- 1 Cup whole farro
- 1 Cup Parmesan cheese, grated
- 4 Tablespoons chopped fresh parsley
- Cooking spray

Procedure:

1. First, spritz the slow cooker with cooking spray.
2. Then, microwave shallots, porcini mushrooms, 1 tablespoon oil, garlic, thyme, ½ teaspoon salt, and ½ teaspoon pepper in a bowl, stirring occasionally, until shallots are softened, about 5 minutes.
3. Now, transfer to the prepared slow cooker.
4. Microwave 2 cups broth and sherry in a separate bowl until steaming, about 5 minutes.
5. Stir broth mixture, cremini mushrooms, and farro into the slow cooker.
6. Cover and cook until farro is tender, 3 to 4 hours on low or 2 to 3 hours on high.
7. Microwave remaining ½ cup broth in a third bowl until steaming, about 2 minutes.
8. Stir broth and Parmesan into farro until the mixture is creamy.
9. Adjust consistency with extra hot broth as needed. Stir in parsley and the remaining 1 tablespoon oil. Season with salt and pepper to taste.
10. Finally, serve.

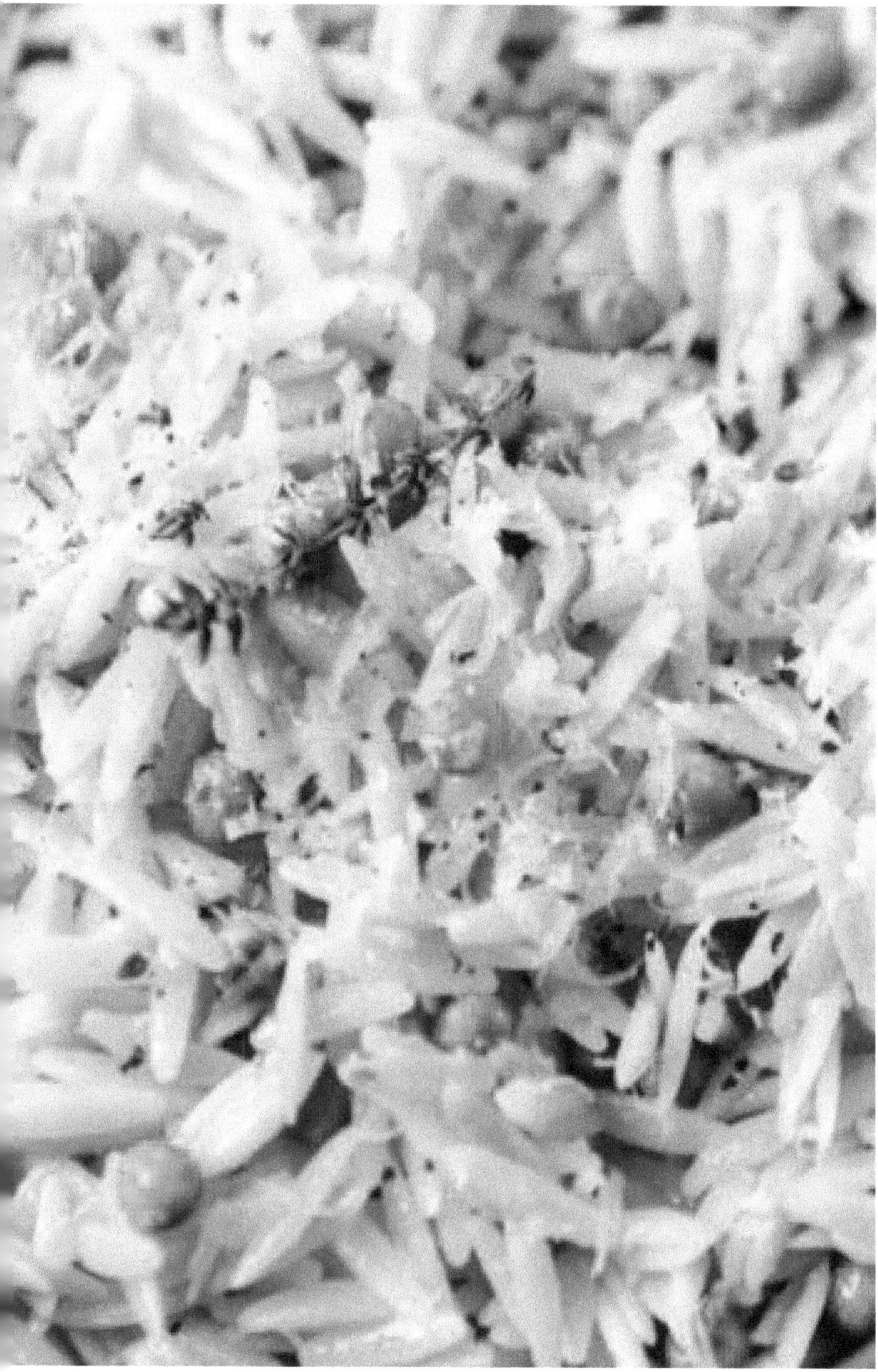

Pleasant Orzo with Peas

Servings: 8

Preparation Time: 2 hours

Ingredients:

- 2 Cups orzo
- 2 Onions, chopped fine
- 12 Garlic cloves, minced
- 6 Tablespoons unsalted butter, divided
- Salt and ground black pepper, to taste
- 5 Cups vegetable or chicken broth, divided, plus extra as needed
- 1/2 Cup dry white wine
- 2 Cups frozen peas, thawed
- 1 Cup parmesan cheese, grated
- 3 Teaspoons grated lemon zest

Procedure:

1. Firstly, microwave orzo, onion, garlic, 1 tablespoon butter, and ½ teaspoon salt in a bowl, stirring occasionally, until orzo is lightly toasted and onion is softened, 5 to 7 minutes. Transfer to the slow cooker.

2. Then, microwave 2 cups broth and wine in a separate bowl until steaming, about 5 minutes.
3. Stir broth mixture into slow cooker, cover, and cook until orzo is al dente, 1 to 2 hours on high.
4. Sprinkle peas over orzo, cover, and let sit until heated through for about 5 minutes.
5. Microwave remaining ½ cup broth in a third bowl until steaming, about 2 minutes.
6. Stir broth, Parmesan, lemon zest, and remaining 2 tablespoons butter into orzo until mixture is creamy. Adjust consistency with extra hot broth as needed.
7. Season with salt and pepper to taste.
8. Finally, serve.

Tasty Tarragon Chicken

Servings: 8

Preparation Time: 3.5 hours

Per Serving: 165 calories, 24.4g protein, 0.6g carbohydrates, 6.5g fat, 0.1g fiber, 73mg cholesterol, 64mg sodium, 448mg potassium.

Ingredients:

- 2-Pounds chicken breast, skinless
- 2 Teaspoons dried tarragon
- 6 Tablespoons lemon juice
- 2 Tablespoons plain yogurt
- 2 Tablespoons olive oil
- 1 Cup of water

Procedure:

1. Firstly, mix olive oil with plain yogurt, lemon juice, and tarragon.
2. Then, brush the chicken breast with tarragon mixture and leave for 10-15 minutes to marinate.

3. After this, pour water in the slow cooker.

4. Now, add chicken breast and close the lid.

5. Finally, cook the chicken on high for 3.5 hours.

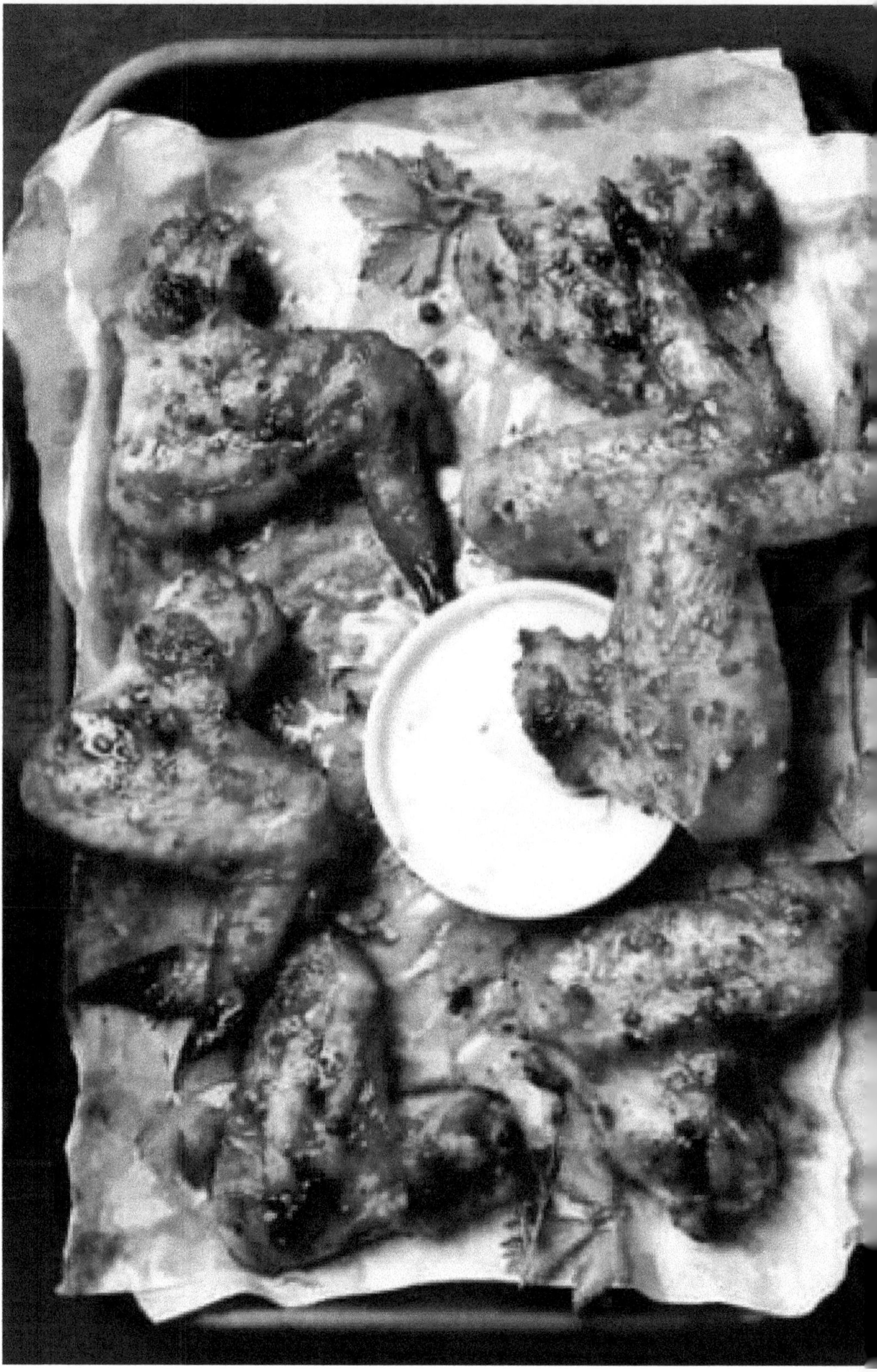

Easy Salsa Chicken Wings

Servings: 10

Preparation Time: 6 hours

Per Serving: 373 calories, 54.1g protein, 6.5g carbohydrates, 13.6g fat, 1.7g fiber, 161mg cholesterol, 781mg sodium, 750mg potassium.

Ingredients:

- 4-Pounds chicken wings
- 4 Cups salsa
- 1 Cup of water

Procedure:

1. Firstly, put all ingredients in the slow cooker.
2. Then, carefully mix the mixture and close the lid.
3. Now, cook the chicken wings on low for 6 hours.

Enjoyable Simple Cheesy Polenta

Servings: 12

Preparation Time: 3 hours

Ingredients:

- 6 Cups water, plus extra as needed
- 2 Cups whole milk
- 2 Cups ground cornmeal
- 4 garlic cloves, minced
- Salt and ground black pepper, to taste
- 1 Cup Parmesan cheese, grated
- 4 Tablespoons unsalted butter
- Cooking spray

Procedure:

1. Firstly, spritz the slow cooker with cooking spray. Whisk water, milk, cornmeal, garlic, and 1 teaspoon salt together in the prepared slow cooker.
2. Then, cover and cook until polenta is tender, 3 to 4 hours on low or 2 to 3 hours on high.

3. Now, whisk Parmesan and butter into polenta until combined.
4. Season with salt and pepper to taste.
5. Finally, serve.

Enticing Quinoa with Corn

Servings: 12

Preparation Time: 3 hours

Ingredients:

- 3 Cups white quinoa, rinsed
- 2 Onions, chopped fine
- 4 Jalapeño chiles, stemmed, deseeded, and minced
- 4 Tablespoons extra-virgin olive oil
- Salt and ground black pepper, to taste
- 3 Cups water
- 2 Cups frozen corn, thawed
- ⅓ Cup minced fresh cilantro
- 4 Tablespoons lime juice
- Cooking spray

Procedure:

1. Firstly, spritz the slow cooker with cooking spray.
2. Then, microwave quinoa, onion, jalapeños, 1 tablespoon oil, and 1 teaspoon salt in a bowl, stirring occasionally, until quinoa is lightly toasted and vegetables are softened for about 5 minutes.

3. Transfer to the prepared slow cooker.

4. Now, stir in water, cover, and cook until quinoa is tender, and all water is absorbed, 3 to 4 hours on low or 2 to 3 hours on high.

5. Sprinkle corn over quinoa, cover, and let sit until heated through for about 5 minutes.

6. Fluff quinoa with fork, then gently folds in cilantro, lime juice, and remaining 1 tablespoon oil.

7. Season with salt and pepper to taste.

8. Finally, serve.

Delightful Orange Chicken

Servings: 8

Preparation Time: 7 hours

Per Serving: 314 calories, 34.9g protein, 24.5g carbohydrates, 8.7g fat, 5.2g fiber, 101mg cholesterol, 101mg sodium, 656mg potassium.

Ingredients:

- 2-Pounds chicken fillet, roughly chopped
- 8 Oranges, peeled, chopped
- 2 Cups of water
- 2 Teaspoons peppercorns
- 2 Onions, diced

Procedure:

1. First, put chicken and oranges in the slow cooker.
2. Then, add water, peppercorns, and onion.
3. Now, close the lid and cook the meal on low for 7 hours.

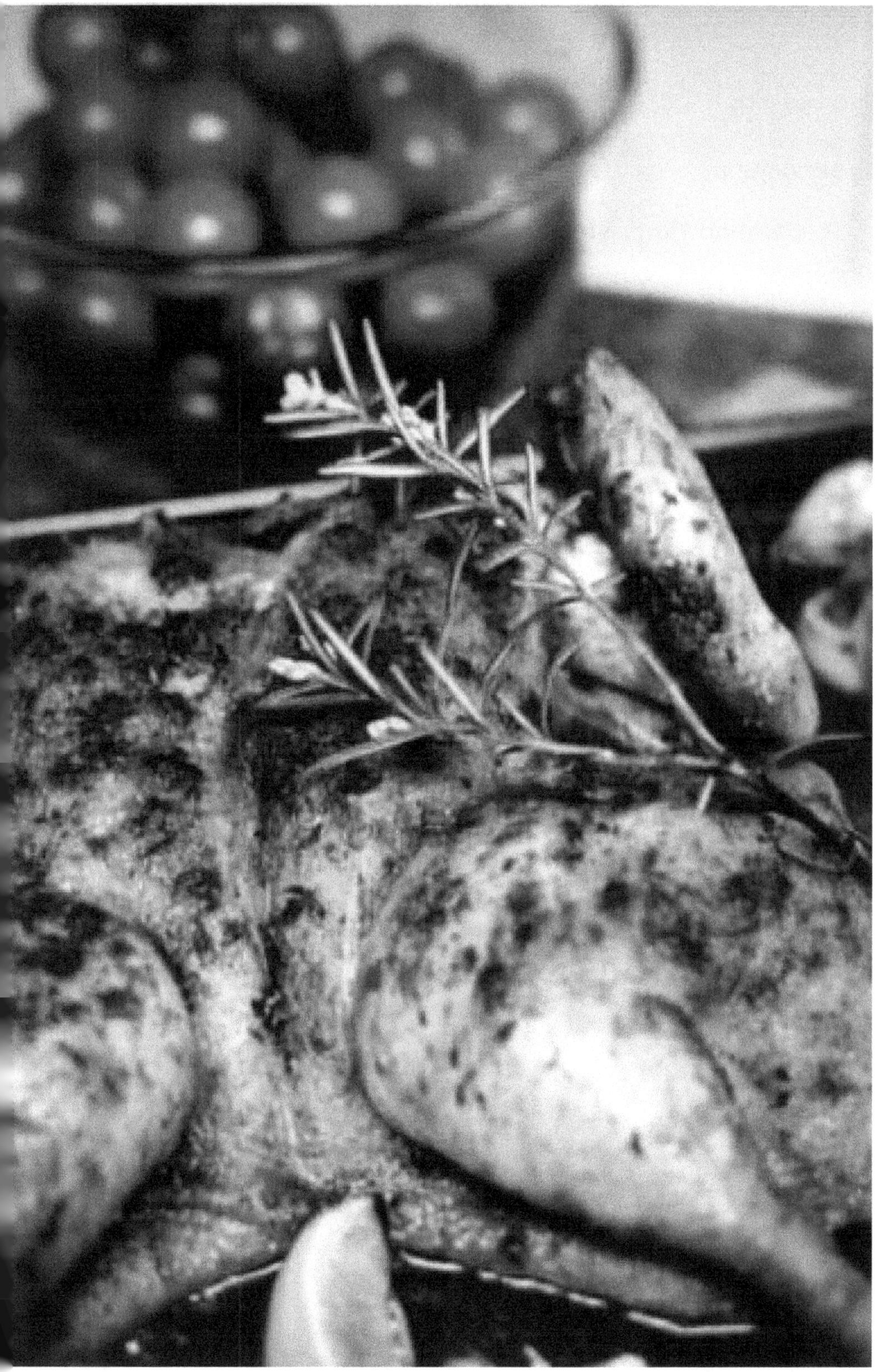

Flavorful Pepper Whole Chicken

Servings: 8

Preparation Time: 8 hours

Per Serving: 254 calories, 33.3g protein, 3.3g carbohydrates, 11.4g fat, 0.8g fiber, 109mg cholesterol, 704mg sodium, 354mg potassium.

Ingredients:

- 32 Oz whole chicken
- 2 Tablespoons ground black pepper
- 2 Teaspoons salt
- 2 Cups bell pepper, chopped
- 4 Cups of water
- 2 Tablespoons butter, softened

Procedure:

1. Firstly, rub the chicken with butter, salt, and ground black pepper.
2. Then, fill it with bell pepper and put it in the slow cooker.
3. Add water and close the lid.
4. Now, cook the chicken on low for 8 hours.

Tasty Italian Style Tenders

Servings: 8

Preparation Time: 3 hours

Per Serving: 202 calories, 24.6g protein, 0.4g carbohydrates, 10.8g fat, 0g fiber, 75mg cholesterol, 657mg sodium, 209mg potassium.

Ingredients:

- 24 Oz chicken fillet
- 1 Tablespoon Italian seasonings
- 1 Cup of water
- 2 Tablespoons olive oil
- 2 Teaspoons salt

Procedure:

1. Firstly, put the chicken into tenders and sprinkle with salt and Italian seasonings.
2. Then, heat the oil in the skillet.
3. Add chicken tenders and cook them on high heat for 1 minute per side.

4. Now, put the chicken tenders in the slow cooker.

5. Add water and close the lid.

6. Finally, cook the chicken for 3 hours on high.

SWEET DISHES

Yummy Double Apple Cake

Servings: 4

Preparation Time: 3 hours

Per Serving: Calories: 235 Fat: 7g Carbs: 40g

Ingredients:

- 1/3 Cup packed dark brown sugar
- Ounces all-purpose flour (about 1 1/2 cups)
- 1/2 Teaspoon baking soda
- 1 Teaspoon ground cinnamon
- ¼ Teaspoon baking powder
- 1/8 Teaspoon salt
- 1/8 Teaspoon ground nutmeg
- 1/8 easpoon ground cloves
- 1/2 Cup unsweetened applesauce
- 1/3 Cup low-fat buttermilk
- 1/8 Cup butter, melted
- 1/2 Tablespoon vanilla extract
- 1/2 Large egg
- 1/2 Cup dried apple slices, coarsely chopped
- 1/2 Teaspoon powdered sugar (optional)

Procedure:

1. Firstly, coat a 5-quart round electric slow cooker with cooking spray.
2. Then, line bottom of slow cooker with parchment paper. Place 2 (30-inch-long) strips of parchment paper in an X pattern under parchment paper liner in slow cooker.
3. Now, coat parchment with cooking spray.
4. Weigh or lightly spoon flour into dry measuring cups; level with a knife.
5. Combine flour, brown sugar, and next 6 ingredients (through to cloves) in a medium bowl, stirring with a whisk.
6. Combine applesauce and next 4 ingredients (through to egg) in a small bowl.
7. Add applesauce mixture to flour mixture, stirring until smooth. Stir in dried apple.
8. Pour batter into prepared slow cooker, spreading into an even layer.
9. Cover and cook on HIGH for 1 to 1 1/2 hours or until puffed and a wooden pick inserted into center comes out clean. Cut into wedges.
10. Finally, sprinkle with powdered sugar, if desired.

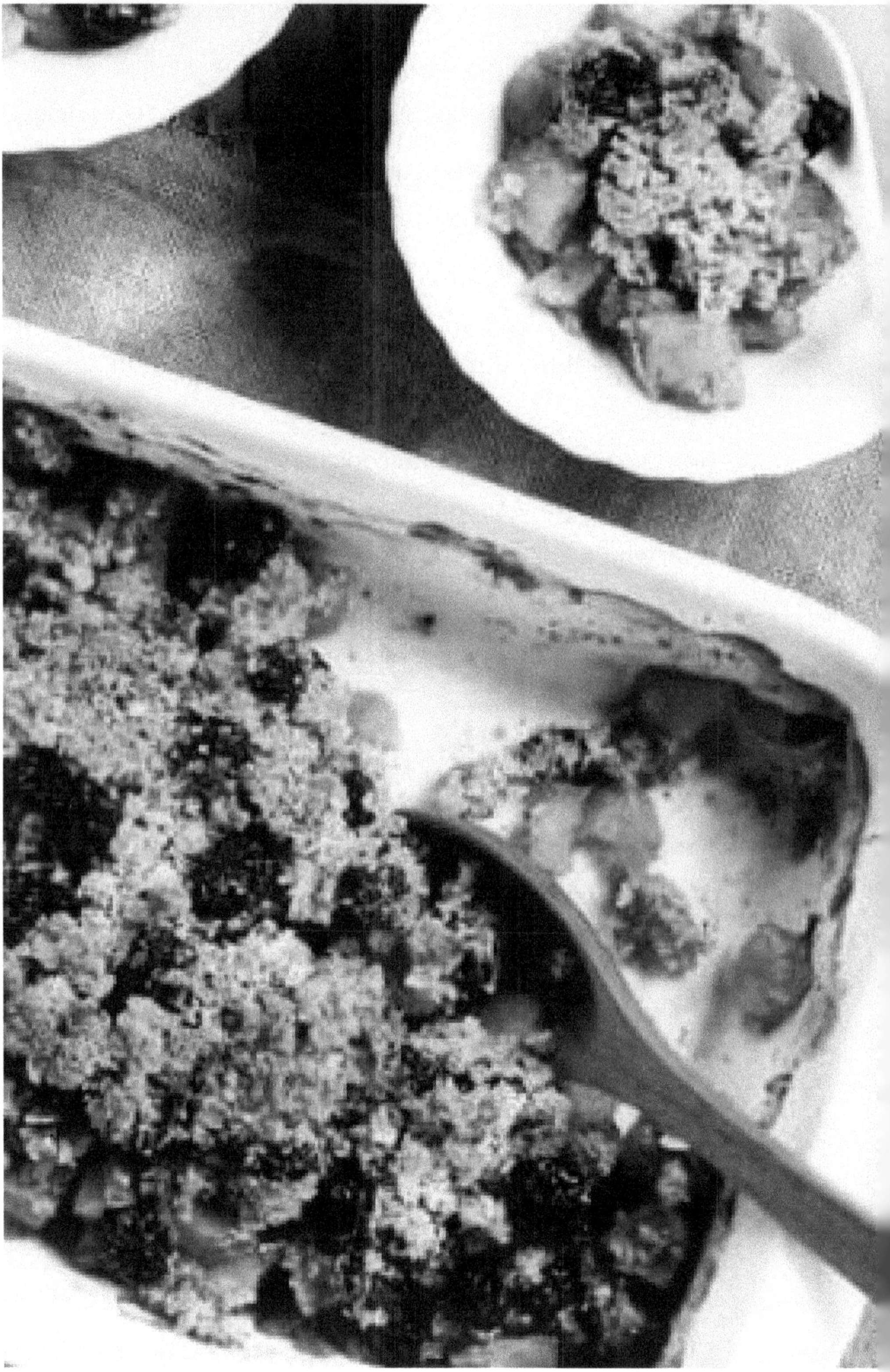

Tasty Blackberry Apple Crisp

Servings: 8

Preparation Time: 3 hours

Per Serving: Calories: 208 Fat: 7g Carbs: 42g

Ingredients:

- 4 Cups organic oats use certified organic
- 1 cup cold butter diced into small pieces or coconut oil
- Optional 1/2 cup nuts of your choice like pecans, walnuts, or almonds
- 4 Tsps cinnamon
- 2 Tsps Chia Seeds
- 2 Tsps of each wheat germ, wheat bran, & oat bran (omit for gluten free)
- 6 Cups Blackberries/Apples or as much as you like/have

Procedure:

1. First, in a medium bowl mix all of the ingredients together except the fruit.
2. Then, fill a 9x5x3 greased loaf pan with the prepared fruit (if your fruit is on the tart side you can sprinkle a

couple of tablespoons of organic sugar over the fruit). Optional: you could also just place your fruit in a greased slow cooker.

3. Top fruit with the oat mixture.
4. Now, place the pan in the slow cooker with no water on the bottom.
5. Finally, slow cook for 1.5 to 2.5 hours on high or 4 hours on low, or until the butter/oil has melted and the fruit is bubbly.

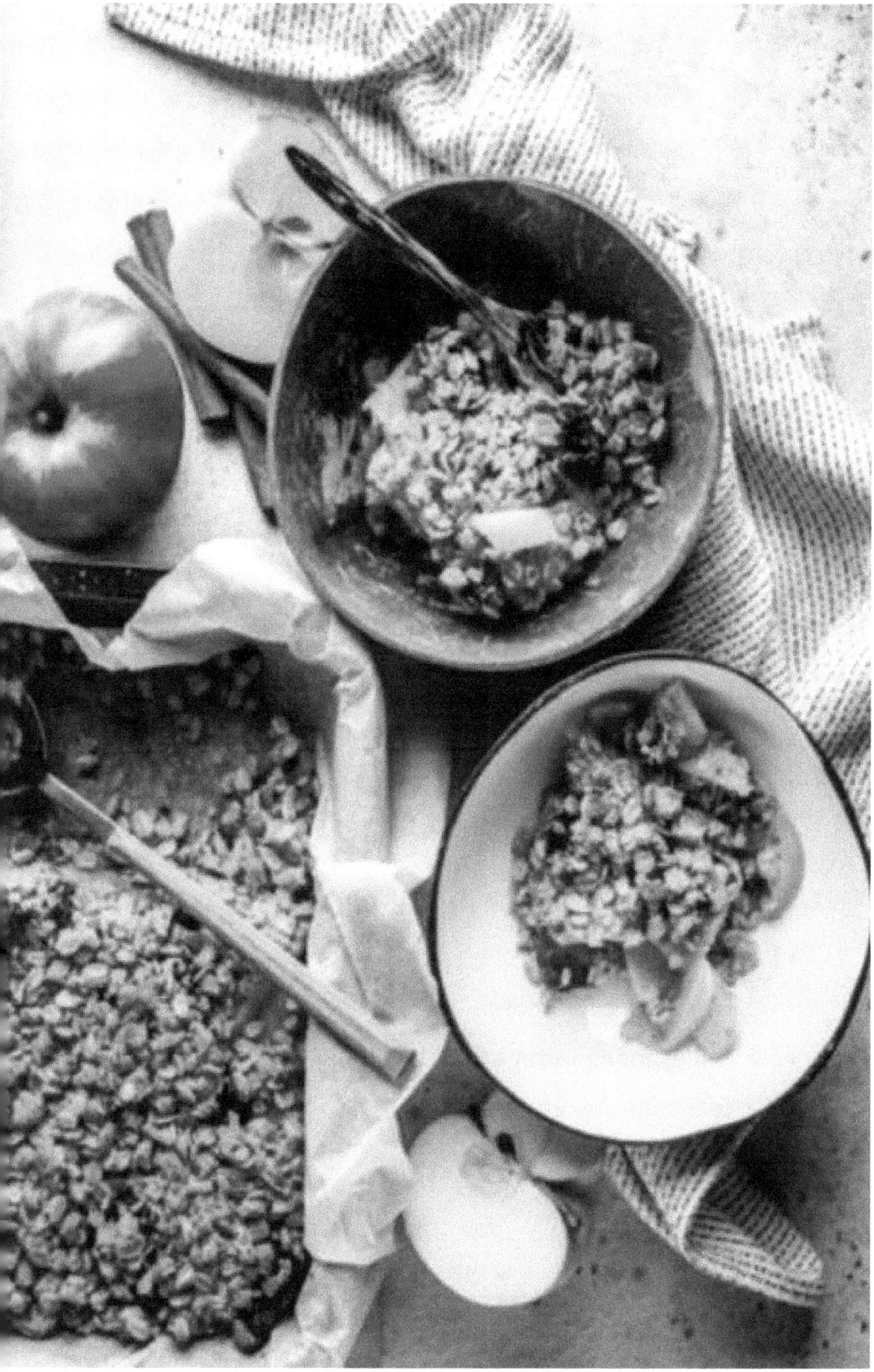

Yummy Caramel Apple Crumble

Servings: 8

Preparation Time: 3 hours

Per Serving: Calories: 190 Fat: 7g Carbs: 32g

Ingredients:

- 2 Cups brown sugar
- 1 Cup granulated sugar
- 10 Large apples, cut into chunks
- 1/8 Teaspoon salt
- 2 Teaspoons cinnamon

Topping

- 2/3 Cup oats
- 2/3 Cup loosely packed brown sugar
- 1/8 Cup flour
- 1 Teaspoon cinnamon
- 2 Tablespoons softened butter
- 2 Teaspoon vanilla extract

Procedure:

1. Firstly, toss apple chunks with salt and cinnamon.
2. Then, in the bottom of your slow-cooker, mix brown and granulated sugars, then spread evenly to cover.
3. Now, layer apples on top, keeping them in a single layer as much as possible, then adding the rest of top.
4. Mix the crumble topping together in a bowl, using your fingers to distribute the butter evenly and thoroughly and clump it together.
5. Sprinkle it over top of the apples.
6. Cook apples on low for 4 hours, or high for 2 hours.
7. Turn off heat, unplug, and let sit, covered, for one hour.
8. During this time the caramel will thicken a bit more.
9. Finally, serve with vanilla ice cream.

Delectable Strawberry Cobbler

Servings: 12

Preparation Time: 3 hours

Per Serving: Calories: 208 Fat: 7g Carbs: 42g

Ingredients:

- 7 lbs strawberries, sliced
- 1 Cup sugar
- 4 Tablespoons cornstarch
- 4 Tablespoons water
- 3/4 Cup brown sugar
- 3/4 Cup quick cooking oats
- 1 Cup flour
- 1 Cup butter

Procedure:

1. Firstly, in a saucepan combine strawberries and regular sugar.
2. Let sit for 30 minutes.
3. Then, after sitting 30 minutes, cook over medium heat for 5 minutes.

4. In a bowl combine cornstarch and water.

5. Stir into berry mixture and bring to a boil.

6. Boil 1 minute or until mixture is thickened.

7. Spoon mixture into slow cooker

8. In a bowl combine brown sugar, oats, and flour.

9. Cut in butter to form a crumbly mixture.

10. Spread evenly over strawberry mixture.

11. Now, cook on low for 2-3 hours.

12. Finally, served warm with ice cream.

Pleasant Triple Chocolate Brownies

Servings: 12

Preparation Time: 3 hours

Per Serving: Calories: 334 Fat: 10g Carbs: 54g

Ingredients:

- 3 Cups all-purpose flour (spooned and leveled)
- 1/2 Cup unsweetened cocoa powder
- 3/4 Teaspoon baking powder
- 1 Teaspoon coarse salt
- 1 Cup (1 stick) unsalted butter, cut into pieces
- 16 Ounces bittersweet chocolate, chopped
- 2 Cups of sugar
- 6 Large eggs, lightly beaten
- 2 Cups of walnut halves, coarsely chopped
- 1 Cup of semisweet chocolate chips (6 ounces)

Procedure:

1. Firstly, lightly coat a 5-quart slow-cooker insert with cooking spray.

2. Line bottom with parchment paper and lightly coat with spray.
3. Then, in a small bowl, whisk together flour, cocoa, baking powder, and salt.
4. Place butter and chocolate in a medium microwave-safe bowl and microwave in 30-second increments, stirring after each, until chocolate is melted.
5. Add sugar; stir to combine. Stir in eggs.
6. Add flour mixture, walnuts, and chocolate chips and stir just until moistened (do not overmix).
7. Transfer to slow cooker and smooth top.
8. Cover and cook on low, 3 1/2 hours. Uncover and cook 30 minutes. Remove insert from slow cooker and run a knife around edge to loosen brownies.
9. Let cool completely in insert on a wire rack, about 2 hours.
10. Finally, turn out onto a work surface and cut into 14 brownies. Store in an airtight container, up to 2 days.

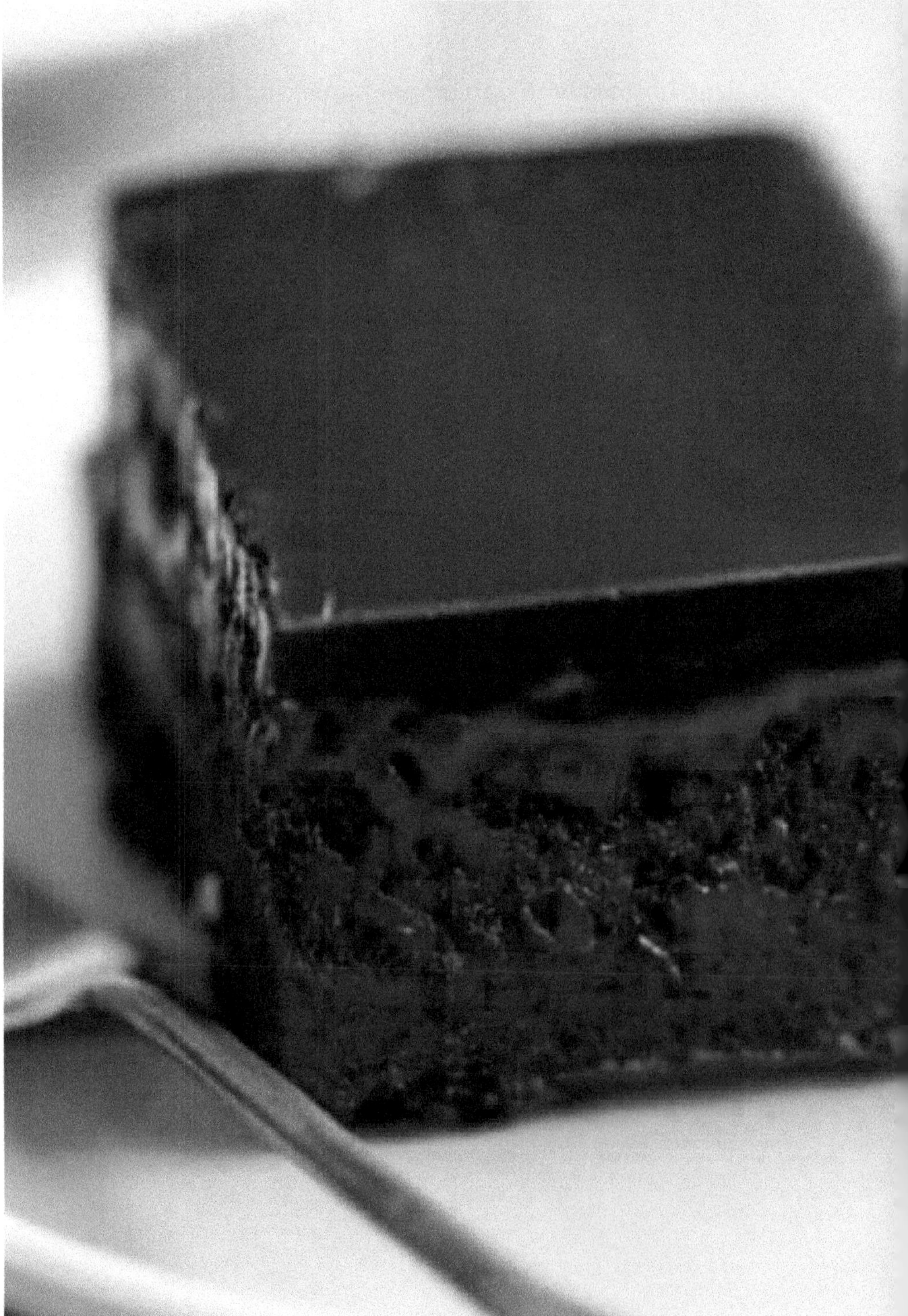

Easy Hot Chocolate Fudge Cake

Servings: 4

Preparation Time: 4 hours

Ingredients:

- 1 Cup packed brown sugar, divided
- 1/2 Cup all-purpose flour
- 3 Tablespoons baking cocoa, divided
- 1 Teaspoon baking powder
- 1/4 Teaspoon salt
- 1/4 Cup 2% milk
- 1Tablespoons butter, melted
- 1/4 Teaspoon vanilla extract
- 1 Cup semisweet chocolate chips
- 1 Cup boiling water
- Vanilla ice cream, for serving
- Cooking spray

Procedure:

1. First, in a bowl, combine 1 cup brown sugar, flour, 3 tablespoons cocoa, baking powder and salt.

2. Combine the milk, butter and vanilla in a separate bowl, stir into dry ingredients just until combined.
3. Then, pour the mixture into the slow cooker coated with cooking spray. Sprinkle with chocolate chips.
4. In a third bowl, combine the remaining brown sugar and cocoa, stir in boiling water. Pour over batter (do not stir).
5. Now, cover and cook on high for 4 to 4½ hours or until a toothpick inserted near center of cake comes out clean.
6. Finally, serve warm with ice cream.

Easy Autumn Apple and Pecan Cake

Servings: 4

Preparation Time: 5 hours

Ingredients:

- 1 (1-pound / 454-g) cans sliced apples, undrained (not pie filling)
- 1/2 (18¼-ounce / 517-g) package spice cake mix
- 1/4 Cup butter, melted
- 1/4 Cup pecans, chopped
- Nonstick cooking spray

Procedure:

1. Firstly, spray the slow cooker with nonstick cooking spray.
2. Then, spoon the apples and their juice into the slow cooker, spreading evenly over the bottom.
3. Sprinkle with spice cake mix.
4. Now, pour the melted butter over the spice cake mix. Top with chopped pecans.
5. Cook on low for 3 to 5 hours, or until a toothpick inserted into topping comes out dry.
6. Finally, serve warm.

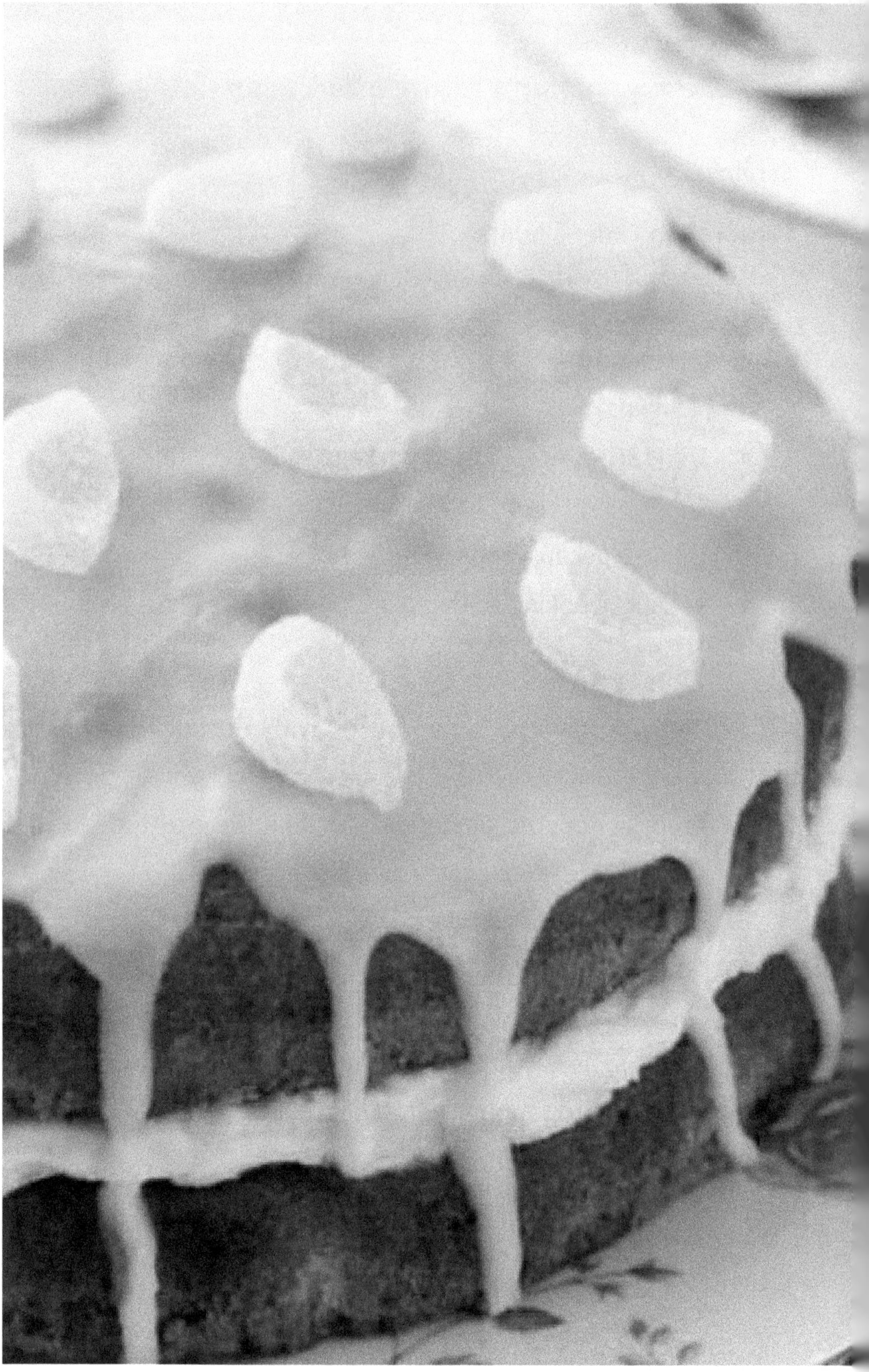

Delightful Simple Lemony Pudding Cake

Servings: 12

Preparation Time: 3 hours

Ingredients:

- 1.1/2 Eggs, whites and yolks separated
- 1/2 Teaspoon lemon zest
- 1/8 Cup lemon juice
- 1.1/2 Tablespoons butter, melted
- 1 Cup milk
- ¾ Cup sugar
- 1/8 Cup flour
- ⅛ Teaspoon salt

Procedure:

1. Firstly, beat the eggs whites until stiff peaks form in a bowl. Set aside.
2. Beat the eggs yolks in a separate bowl.
3. Then, blend in the lemon zest, lemon juice, butter, and milk.
4. In a third bowl, combine the sugar, flour, and salt.

5. Now, add to the egg-lemon mixture, beating until smooth.
6. Fold them into the beaten egg whites. Spoon the mixture into the slow cooker.
7. Cover and cook on high for 2 to 3 hours.

Delicious Apple Cake with Walnut

Servings: 5

Preparation Time: 4 hours

Ingredients:

- 1 Cup sugar
- 1/2 Cup olive oil
- 1 Egg
- 1/2 Teaspoon vanilla
- 1 Cup chopped apples
- 1 Cup flour
- 1/2 Teaspoon salt
- 1/2 Teaspoon baking soda
- 1/2 Teaspoon nutmeg
- 1/2 Cup chopped walnuts

Procedure:

1. First, beat together the sugar, oil, and eggs in a large bowl. Add vanilla and apples. Mix well.
2. Sift together flour, salt, baking soda, and nutmeg in a bowl.

3. Then, add dry ingredients and nuts to the apple mixture. Stir well.
4. Pour batter into greased and floured cake pan that fits into the slow cooker.
5. Cover with pan's lid or greased foil.
6. Place pan in the slow cooker. Cover cooker.
7. Bake on high for 3½ to 4 hours. Let cake stand in pan for 5 minutes after removing from the slow cooker.
8. Finally, remove the cake from pan, slice and serve.

Delectable Peach Bread Pudding

Servings: 12

Preparation Time: 6 hours

Per Serving: 181 calories, 4.2g protein, 18.1g carbohydrates, 10.4g fat, 0.8g fiber, 82mg cholesterol, 189mg sodium, 82mg potassium.

Ingredients:

- 10 Oz white bread, chopped
- 4 Eggs, beaten
- 2 Cups heavy cream
- 1 Cup peaches, chopped
- 2 Teaspoons flour
- 2 Teaspoons coconut oil
- 4 Tablespoons sugar

Procedure:

1. Firstly, grease the slow cooker bottom with coconut oil.
2. Then, add white bread.

3. Mix heavy cream with eggs, flour, sugar, and pour over the bread.
4. Now, add peaches and close the lid.
5. Finally, cook the pudding on low for 6 hours.

Flavorful Almond Bars

Servings: 12

Preparation Time: 2 hours

Per Serving: 266 calories, 6.4g protein, 26g carbohydrates, 16.5g fat, 5.8g fiber, 55mg cholesterol, 22mg sodium, 206mg potassium.

Ingredients:

- 2 Tablespoons cocoa powder
- 1 Cup flour
- 1 Cup coconut flour
- 8 Tablespoons coconut oil
- 2 Teaspoons baking powder
- 4 Oz almonds, chopped
- 1/2 Cup of sugar
- 4 Eggs, beaten

Procedure:

1. Firstly, mix all ingredients in the bowl and knead the smooth dough.

2. The put the dough in the slow cooker, flatten it, and cut into bars.

3. Then, close the lid and cook the dessert on high for 2 hours.

Easy Pineapple upside Down Cake

Servings: 4

Preparation Time: 2.5 hours

Per Serving: 205 calories, 5.8g protein, 29.8g carbohydrates, 7.1g fat, 0.9g fiber, 95mg cholesterol, 70mg sodium, 148mg potassium.

Ingredients:

- 1/4 Cup milk
- 1.1/2 Tablespoons butter, melted
- 2 Eggs, beaten
- 1/3 Cup sugar
- 1/2 Teaspoon vanilla extract
- 1 Cup flour
- 2.1/2 Oz pineapple, sliced
- 1/2 Teaspoon baking powder

Procedure:

1. Firstly, in the bowl, mix milk, butter, eggs, vanilla extract, sugar, and flour.

2. Then, add baking powder and mix the mixture until you get a smooth batter.
3. After this, line the slow cooker with baking paper.
4. Now, put the sliced pineapples in the slow cooker in one layer.
5. Pour the batter over the pineapples and close the lid.
6. Finally, cook the cake on high for 2.5 hours.